Foreword

In the tender years of our lives, our parents are our guiding lights, our pillars of strength, and our unwavering source of love. As we journey through life, their roles evolve, and inevitably, the time comes when the hands that once held ours now need our support in return.

"Tender Care at Sunset" is not just a book; it's a heartfelt ode to the intricate dance of life, where roles reverse, and the circle of care completes itself. In these pages, you'll find a treasure trove of wisdom, compassion, and practical guidance for navigating the delicate terrain of supporting aging parents with love, understanding, and dignity.

Caring for aging parents is a journey filled with both tender moments and profound challenges. It's a journey that tests our patience, stretches our empathy, and deepens our capacity for love.

From understanding the intricacies of the aging process to navigating complex family dynamics, "Tender Care at Sunset" offers a comprehensive roadmap for every stage of the caregiving journey. You'll learn essential caregiving skills, explore strategies for promoting emotional well-being, and gain invaluable insights into navigating the financial, legal, and end-of-life aspects of care.

But perhaps most importantly, this book is a gentle reminder of the importance of preserving the dignity and autonomy of our aging loved ones. It's a call to action to embrace the inherent worth and wisdom of those who have shaped our lives and to honor their legacy with grace and respect.

As you embark on this journey of caregiving, may "Tender Care at Sunset" serve as your trusted companion, offering solace in moments of doubt, guidance in moments of uncertainty, and inspiration in moments of weariness. May it remind you that while the road ahead may be challenging, it is also profoundly meaningful—a testament to the enduring power of love and the resilience of the human spirit.

So, with an open heart and a willing spirit, let us embark together on this sacred journey of caring for our aging parents—guided by love, fueled by compassion, and anchored in the unwavering belief that every tender moment of care is a testament to the depth of our love and the richness of our humanity.

Table of Contents

Chapter 1: Understanding Aging and Its Challenges

1.1 Introduction to the Aging Process

Aging is a universal and inevitable process that all living organisms experience. It is a complex phenomenon marked by a gradual decline in physiological function and an increased susceptibility to disease and disability. While aging is often associated with negative connotations, it is essential to recognize that it is also a natural and integral part of the human experience. By understanding the aging process more deeply, we can better appreciate the challenges faced by older adults and develop more effective strategies for supporting them with love, understanding, and dignity.

The aging process is characterized by a myriad of physiological changes that occur at the cellular, tissue, and organ levels. One of the most notable changes is the gradual decline in organ function, including the heart, lungs, kidneys, and brain. For example, the cardiovascular system undergoes changes such as decreased elasticity of blood vessels and reduced cardiac output, leading to conditions like hypertension and heart disease. Similarly, the respiratory system experiences a decline in lung function, making older adults more vulnerable to respiratory infections and diseases such as chronic obstructive pulmonary disease (COPD).

At the cellular level, aging is accompanied by a phenomenon known as cellular senescence, where cells lose their ability to divide and replicate. This contributes to the accumulation of damaged DNA and proteins, leading to a decline in tissue repair and regeneration. Additionally, oxidative stress and inflammation play significant roles in the aging process, contributing to the development of age-related diseases such as cancer, Alzheimer's disease, and osteoarthritis.

In addition to physiological changes, aging also brings about psychological changes that can impact mental health and well-being. One common psychological challenge faced by older adults is cognitive decline, which can manifest as difficulties with memory, attention, and executive function. While some degree of cognitive decline is a normal part of aging, severe impairments can significantly impact daily functioning and quality of life.

Another psychological challenge associated with aging is the increased prevalence of mental health disorders such as depression and anxiety. Older adults may experience losses such as the death of loved ones, retirement, and declining health, which can contribute to feelings of sadness, loneliness, and hopelessness. Furthermore, social isolation and loneliness are significant risk factors for poor mental health outcomes in older adults, highlighting the importance of fostering social connections and support networks.

In addition to physiological and psychological changes, aging also brings about significant social changes that can influence the well-being of older adults. One of the most significant social changes associated with aging is the transition from the workforce to retirement. While retirement can provide opportunities for leisure and relaxation, it can also lead to feelings of purposelessness and loss of identity for some individuals.

Furthermore, aging often entails changes in social roles and relationships, including the loss of spouses, friends, and family members. This can result in feelings of loneliness and social isolation, which are associated with adverse health outcomes such as depression, cognitive decline, and mortality. Additionally, older adults may face ageism and discrimination in various domains of life, including employment, healthcare, and social interactions, which can further exacerbate feelings of marginalization and exclusion.

The aging process is a multifaceted phenomenon that encompasses physiological, psychological, and social changes. While aging is often accompanied by challenges such as physical decline, cognitive impairment, and social isolation, it is essential to recognize that older adults also possess strengths, resilience, and wisdom accumulated over a lifetime of experiences. By understanding the complexities of the aging process more deeply, we can develop more compassionate and effective approaches to supporting older adults with love, understanding, and dignity. Ultimately, aging is not just a process of decline; it is also a journey of growth, transformation, and continued contributions to society.

1.2 Common Physical and Cognitive Changes in Aging

Aging is a natural and inevitable process that all individuals undergo as they progress through the various stages of life. It is marked by a multitude of physical, cognitive, and psychosocial changes that occur gradually over time. While aging is a normal part of the human experience, it is essential to recognize and understand the challenges associated with these changes, both for the individuals experiencing them and for the caregivers and healthcare professionals who support them.

Physical Changes

As individuals age, they experience a myriad of physical changes that affect nearly every system in the body. These changes can impact older adults' mobility, sensory perception, and overall functional independence. Understanding these changes is crucial for identifying age-related health risks and implementing appropriate interventions to support older adults' well-being.

1. Musculoskeletal Changes: One of the most noticeable physical changes associated with aging is the loss of muscle mass and strength, a condition known as sarcopenia. Sarcopenia can lead to decreased mobility, increased risk of falls, and diminished quality of life for older adults. Additionally, changes in bone density and structure, such as osteopenia and osteoporosis, increase the risk of fractures and bone injuries in older adults.

2. Sensory Changes: Aging also affects sensory perception, including vision, hearing, taste, and smell. Visual acuity declines with age, leading to difficulties with reading, driving, and navigating the environment. Similarly, age-related hearing loss, known as presbycusis, can impair communication and social interaction for older adults. Changes in taste and smell perception can affect older adults' appetite and nutritional intake, potentially leading to malnutrition and other health problems.

3. Cardiovascular Changes: The cardiovascular system undergoes significant changes with aging, including decreased elasticity of blood vessels, reduced cardiac output, and increased arterial stiffness. These changes can contribute to hypertension, atherosclerosis, and other cardiovascular diseases that are common among older adults. Additionally, older adults are at increased risk of developing heart failure, arrhythmias, and other cardiac conditions as a result of age-related changes in cardiac structure and function.

4. Respiratory Changes: Aging also affects respiratory function, leading to changes such as decreased lung elasticity, reduced lung capacity, and diminished respiratory muscle strength. These changes can impair older adults' ability to effectively exchange oxygen and carbon dioxide, leading to respiratory conditions such as chronic obstructive pulmonary disease (COPD), pneumonia, and respiratory failure.

Cognitive Changes

In addition to physical changes, aging is also associated with cognitive changes that can affect older adults' memory, attention, and executive function. While some degree of cognitive decline is a normal part of aging, severe impairments can significantly impact older adults' daily functioning and quality of life. Understanding these cognitive changes is essential for identifying cognitive impairment and implementing appropriate interventions to support older adults' cognitive health and well-being.

1. Memory Changes: One of the most common cognitive changes associated with aging is changes in memory function. Older adults may experience difficulties with episodic memory, which involves recalling past events and experiences. They may also experience challenges with working memory, which involves holding and manipulating information in the mind for short periods. While some memory decline is normal with aging, severe impairments in memory function may indicate the presence of a neurodegenerative condition such as Alzheimer's disease or other forms of dementia.

2. Attention and Processing Speed: Aging can also affect older adults' attention and processing speed, leading to difficulties with tasks that require sustained attention and rapid information processing. Older adults may take longer to complete cognitive tasks and may have difficulty filtering out irrelevant information in complex environments. These changes can impact older adults' ability to perform activities of daily living, engage in social interactions, and maintain independence.

3. Executive Function: Executive function refers to a set of cognitive processes involved in planning, problem-solving, decision-making, and self-regulation. Aging can affect older adults' executive function, leading to difficulties with tasks such as organizing, prioritizing, and multitasking. Older adults may experience challenges with inhibitory control, which involves suppressing irrelevant or distracting information, as well as difficulties with cognitive flexibility, which involves adapting to changing task demands and shifting between different cognitive processes.

The physical and cognitive changes associated with aging have significant implications for older adults' health, well-being, and quality of life. Older adults may experience limitations in mobility, sensory perception, and overall functional independence as a result of age-related physical changes. Additionally, cognitive changes such as memory decline, attention deficits, and executive dysfunction can impair older adults' ability to perform daily tasks, engage in social interactions, and maintain independence.

Understanding these changes is crucial for identifying age-related health risks, implementing appropriate interventions, and providing support to older adults as they navigate the challenges of aging. Healthcare professionals and caregivers must work collaboratively to develop comprehensive and person-centered approaches to supporting older adults' health and well-being. This may involve implementing strategies to promote physical activity, prevent falls, and optimize nutritional intake to address age-related physical changes. It may also involve providing cognitive stimulation, social engagement, and emotional support to address age-related cognitive changes and promote cognitive health.

The physical and cognitive changes associated with aging are complex and multifaceted phenomena that have significant implications for older adults' health, well-being, and quality of life. Understanding these changes is essential for identifying age-related health risks, implementing appropriate interventions, and providing support to older adults as they navigate the challenges of aging. By developing a deeper understanding of the physical and cognitive changes associated with aging, healthcare professionals and caregivers can work collaboratively to promote healthy aging and enhance the quality of life for older adults around the world.

1.3 Emotional and Psychological Impact of Aging

Aging is a multifaceted process that encompasses not only physical changes but also emotional and psychological transformations. As individuals progress through the various stages of life, they encounter a myriad of emotional and psychological challenges that can profoundly impact their well-being and quality of life. By understanding these complexities, we can develop more compassionate and effective approaches to supporting older adults as they navigate the joys and challenges of aging.

Emotional Resilience and Adaptation

One of the key themes that emerge when considering the emotional and psychological impact of aging is the concept of resilience and adaptation. While aging inevitably brings about changes and challenges, many older adults demonstrate remarkable resilience in the face of adversity. Research has shown that older adults often report higher levels of emotional well-being and life satisfaction compared to younger adults, a phenomenon known as the "paradox of aging."

One explanation for this paradox is the theory of emotional selectivity, which suggests that as individuals age, they become more selective in their choice of social partners and activities, focusing on those that are most emotionally meaningful and rewarding. This selective focus on positive experiences may contribute to older adults' enhanced emotional well-being and satisfaction with life.

Additionally, older adults often develop a sense of acceptance and wisdom that allows them to navigate life's challenges with greater equanimity and grace. They may draw on their life experiences and accumulated wisdom to cope with adversity, finding meaning and purpose in the face of difficult circumstances. Furthermore, older adults may cultivate a greater sense of gratitude and appreciation for life's blessings, fostering a positive outlook and resilience in the face of adversity.

However, it is essential to recognize that not all older adults experience emotional resilience and adaptation in the same way. Many older adults face significant emotional and psychological challenges, including grief and loss, loneliness and social isolation, and mental health disorders such as depression and anxiety. Understanding these challenges is crucial for providing appropriate support and interventions to promote emotional well-being and quality of life for older adults.

Grief and Loss

One of the most significant emotional challenges associated with aging is the experience of grief and loss. As individuals age, they inevitably encounter losses such as the death of loved ones, the loss of physical health and independence, and the loss of social roles and identities. These losses can evoke a range of emotions, including sadness, anger, guilt, and despair, which may impact older adults' emotional well-being and quality of life.

Grief is a natural and normal response to loss, and it is essential for older adults to allow themselves to grieve and process their emotions in their own time and way. However, unresolved grief or prolonged mourning can contribute to feelings of depression, anxiety, and hopelessness, which may require professional intervention and support.

It is also important to recognize that grief is not limited to the death of loved ones but can also encompass other types of losses, such as the loss of physical health and functional independence. Older adults may experience grief and mourning as they navigate the challenges of aging, including chronic illness, disability, and changes in living arrangements and social support networks.

Loneliness and Social Isolation

Another significant emotional challenge faced by many older adults is loneliness and social isolation. As individuals age, they may experience changes in their social networks and support systems, including the loss of friends and family members, retirement from work, and physical limitations that restrict their ability to engage in social activities and maintain social connections.

Loneliness and social isolation can have profound implications for older adults' emotional well-being and mental health. Research has shown that loneliness is associated with a range of adverse health outcomes, including depression, anxiety, cognitive decline, and increased mortality risk. Additionally, social isolation can exacerbate existing health problems and reduce older adults' access to essential support services and resources.

Addressing loneliness and social isolation requires a multifaceted approach that encompasses both individual and community-level interventions. Older adults may benefit from interventions aimed at enhancing social support networks, fostering social connections, and promoting community engagement and participation. Additionally, healthcare professionals and caregivers can work collaboratively to implement programs and services that address the social determinants of health and promote social inclusion and connectedness for older adults.

Mental Health Disorders

In addition to grief and loneliness, many older adults also experience mental health disorders such as depression and anxiety. While mental health disorders are not a normal part of aging, they are more common among older adults compared to younger age groups, and they can have significant implications for older adults' emotional well-being and quality of life.

Depression is one of the most common mental health disorders among older adults, affecting millions of older adults worldwide. It is characterized by persistent feelings of sadness, hopelessness, and worthlessness, as well as changes in appetite, sleep, and energy levels. Depression can significantly impact older adults' functioning and quality of life, impairing their ability to perform daily activities, engage in social interactions, and maintain relationships.

Anxiety is another common mental health disorder among older adults, characterized by excessive worry, fear, and apprehension about future events or situations. Anxiety disorders can manifest in various forms, including generalized anxiety disorder, panic disorder, phobias, and obsessive-compulsive disorder. Like depression, anxiety can have significant implications for older adults' emotional well-being and quality of life, interfering with their ability to function and engage in meaningful activities.

The emotional and psychological impact of aging is a complex and multifaceted phenomenon that encompasses a range of experiences, challenges, and opportunities. While aging inevitably brings about changes and losses, many older adults demonstrate remarkable resilience in the face of adversity, drawing on their life experiences and accumulated wisdom to navigate life's challenges with grace and dignity. However, it is essential to recognize that not all older adults experience emotional resilience and adaptation in the same way, and many face significant emotional and psychological challenges, including grief and loss, loneliness and social isolation, and mental health disorders such as depression and anxiety.

Understanding these challenges is crucial for providing appropriate support and interventions to promote emotional well-being and quality of life for older adults. By addressing the emotional and psychological needs of older adults in a compassionate and person-centered manner, we can enhance their resilience, foster their well-being, and ensure that they continue to thrive and flourish as they age.

1.4 Challenges Faced by Aging Parents and Their Families

As individuals age, they encounter a myriad of physical, emotional, and social changes that can have profound implications for their well-being and quality of life. These changes often bring about a host of challenges for aging parents and their families, as they navigate the complexities of providing care and support to their loved ones. By understanding these challenges, we can develop more compassionate and effective approaches to supporting aging parents and their families as they navigate the journey of aging together.

Financial Challenges

One of the most significant challenges faced by aging parents and their families is financial strain. As individuals age, they may experience a decline in income and financial resources, particularly if they are retired or no longer able to work due to health-related issues. Additionally, older adults may face increased expenses associated with healthcare, long-term care, and other essential needs, placing a significant burden on both the aging parents and their families.

For many families, the financial challenges associated with aging can be overwhelming, particularly if they are already struggling to make ends meet. Older adults may feel anxious and uncertain about their financial future, while their families may experience stress and worry about how to afford the cost of care and support services. Additionally, financial strain can strain family relationships, leading to conflict and tension among family members as they struggle to navigate the complexities of financial decision-making and resource allocation.

Addressing financial challenges requires a multifaceted approach that encompasses both individual and systemic interventions. Older adults may benefit from financial planning and management services aimed at helping them budget, save, and invest their resources effectively. Additionally, families may benefit from access to financial assistance programs and resources that can help alleviate the financial burden of caregiving and long-term care.

Caregiving Responsibilities

Another significant challenge faced by aging parents and their families is the responsibility of providing care and support to older adults as they age. Many families find themselves thrust into the role of caregiver, assuming primary responsibility for meeting their aging parents' physical, emotional, and social needs. While caregiving can be a rewarding and fulfilling experience, it can also be emotionally and physically demanding, particularly if the caregiver is balancing caregiving responsibilities with other roles and obligations, such as work, parenting, and personal life.

Caregiving can take a toll on caregivers' mental and physical health, leading to stress, burnout, and exhaustion. Caregivers may experience feelings of guilt, resentment, and overwhelm as they struggle to meet their aging parents' needs while also managing their own well-being. Additionally, caregiving responsibilities can strain family relationships, leading to conflict and tension among family members as they navigate the complexities of caregiving decision-making and coordination.

Addressing caregiving challenges requires a comprehensive and collaborative approach that involves both individual and systemic interventions. Caregivers may benefit from access to respite care services, support groups, and counseling to help them cope with the emotional and physical demands of caregiving. Additionally, families may benefit from access to community-based support services and resources that can help alleviate the burden of caregiving and provide assistance with tasks such as transportation, meal preparation, and household chores.

Healthcare and Long-Term Care

Aging parents and their families also face challenges related to accessing healthcare and long-term care services. As individuals age, they may experience an increased need for medical care and support, particularly if they are managing chronic health conditions or disabilities. Additionally, older adults may require assistance with activities of daily living, such as bathing, dressing, and medication management, which can be difficult for families to provide on their own.

Accessing healthcare and long-term care services can be challenging for aging parents and their families, particularly if they are navigating complex healthcare systems and insurance networks. Older adults may face barriers to accessing care, such as limited transportation, mobility issues, and financial constraints, which can prevent them from receiving the care and support they need to maintain their health and independence.

Addressing healthcare and long-term care challenges requires a coordinated and collaborative approach that involves both individual and systemic interventions. Older adults may benefit from access to comprehensive healthcare services, including preventive care, chronic disease management, and rehabilitation services. Additionally, families may benefit from access to long-term care options, such as home health care, assisted living, and nursing home care, that can provide support and assistance with activities of daily living.

Aging parents and their families face a myriad of challenges as they navigate the complexities of aging together. From financial strain to caregiving responsibilities to accessing healthcare and long-term care services, the challenges of aging are multifaceted. However, by understanding these challenges and working collaboratively to address them, aging parents and their families can overcome adversity and build resilience in the face of aging. By developing more compassionate and effective approaches to supporting aging parents and their families, we can ensure that older adults are able to age with dignity, independence, and quality of life.

Chapter 2: Building Empathy and Compassion

2.1 Developing Empathy for Aging Parents

Empathy is a fundamental aspect of human connection and understanding, allowing individuals to perceive and understand the experiences, emotions, and perspectives of others. It plays a crucial role in building strong relationships, fostering compassion, and promoting mutual support and understanding. When it comes to aging parents, developing empathy is particularly important, as it enables adult children to connect with their parents on a deeper level, appreciate their unique experiences and challenges, and provide meaningful support and care.

Before delving into the specifics of developing empathy for aging parents, it's essential to understand the nature of aging itself. Aging is a natural and inevitable process that encompasses a myriad of physical, emotional, and social changes. These changes can be challenging and often evoke a range of emotions, including fear, sadness, frustration, and uncertainty.

It's important to recognize that aging is not a uniform experience—each individual's journey through aging is unique, shaped by a variety of factors such as genetics, lifestyle, socioeconomic status, and personal history. Additionally, aging is not a static process—it evolves over time, influenced by both internal and external factors. By understanding the complexities of aging and appreciating the diversity of experiences within the aging population, adult children can develop greater empathy and sensitivity towards their aging parents' needs, preferences, and challenges.

The Importance of Empathy for Aging Parents

Empathy is a cornerstone of effective communication and relationship-building, particularly in the context of caregiving and support for aging parents. When adult children cultivate empathy for their aging parents, they are better able to:

1. Understand their parents' perspectives and experiences: Empathy allows adult children to see the world through their aging parents' eyes, appreciating the challenges they face and the emotions they experience. By empathizing with their parents' perspectives, adult children can gain insight into their needs, preferences, and values, guiding them in providing more meaningful and personalized support and care.

2. Validate their parents' emotions and feelings: Aging can be a time of profound change and transition, often accompanied by a rollercoaster of emotions. When adult children empathize with their aging parents' feelings—whether it's fear, sadness, frustration, or joy—they create a safe and supportive space for their parents to express themselves authentically. Validating their parents' emotions helps strengthen the parent-child bond and fosters a sense of trust and connection.

3. Offer emotional support and comfort: Empathy enables adult children to offer emotional support and comfort to their aging parents during times of distress or difficulty. By empathizing with

their parents' emotions and providing a listening ear, adult children can help alleviate feelings of loneliness, anxiety, or sadness, fostering emotional well-being and resilience in their parents.

4. Foster collaboration and decision-making: When adult children empathize with their aging parents' perspectives and experiences, they are more likely to engage in collaborative decision-making and problem-solving. Empathy facilitates open communication, mutual understanding, and respectful dialogue, enabling families to navigate complex issues and challenges together with compassion and empathy.

Practical Strategies for Cultivating Empathy

Developing empathy for aging parents is an ongoing process that requires intention, practice, and reflection. Here are some practical strategies for cultivating empathy and enhancing communication and connection with aging parents:

1. Practice active listening: Active listening involves fully focusing on and understanding what the other person is saying, without interrupting or judging. When interacting with aging parents, adult children can practice active listening by giving their full attention, maintaining eye contact, and paraphrasing their parents' words to demonstrate understanding and empathy.

2. Ask open-ended questions: Open-ended questions encourage aging parents to share their thoughts, feelings, and experiences more freely, facilitating deeper conversation and connection. Adult children can ask questions such as "How are you feeling today?" or

"What has been on your mind lately?" to invite their parents to express themselves and share their perspectives.

3. Validate emotions and feelings: Validation involves acknowledging and accepting the legitimacy of another person's emotions and feelings, even if they differ from our own. When aging parents express emotions such as sadness, frustration, or fear, adult children can validate their parents' feelings by saying things like "I understand why you might feel that way" or "It's okay to feel upset about this."

4. Practice perspective-taking: Perspective-taking involves imagining oneself in another person's shoes, seeing the world from their point of view, and understanding their thoughts, feelings, and experiences. Adult children can practice perspective-taking by reflecting on their aging parents' life experiences, challenges, and values, and considering how these factors influence their parents' perspectives and behaviors.

5. Show empathy through gestures and actions: Empathy is not only conveyed through words but also through gestures, actions, and nonverbal cues. Adult children can show empathy towards their aging parents by offering physical affection, spending quality time together, and providing practical support with tasks such as grocery shopping, household chores, or transportation.

6. Seek support and education: Developing empathy for aging parents can be challenging, particularly if adult children have limited experience or understanding of aging-related issues. Adult children can seek support and education from resources such as books,

articles, support groups, and workshops focused on aging, caregiving, and communication skills. Learning from others' experiences and perspectives can enhance empathy and provide valuable insights and strategies for supporting aging parents.

Developing empathy for aging parents is a transformative and rewarding journey that deepens the bond between adult children and their parents, fosters mutual understanding and support, and enhances the quality of life for both generations. By understanding the complexities of aging, appreciating the diversity of experiences within the aging population, and practicing empathy in their interactions with their aging parents, adult children can create a compassionate and supportive environment that honors their parents' dignity, autonomy, and well-being.

As aging parents and their families navigate the challenges and opportunities of aging together, empathy serves as a guiding light, illuminating the path towards deeper connection, meaningful communication, and shared understanding.

2.2 Understanding the Importance of Compassionate Care

Caring for aging parents is a profound and complex responsibility that many individuals face as their parents grow older and require assistance with daily activities, medical care, and emotional support. Providing compassionate care for aging parents goes beyond meeting their physical needs—it involves fostering emotional connection, promoting dignity and respect, and honoring their autonomy and independence.

As individuals age, they may experience a range of physical, emotional, and social changes that impact their well-being and quality of life. From declining physical health and mobility to changes in cognitive function and sensory perception, aging brings about unique challenges and vulnerabilities for older adults. Additionally, aging is often accompanied by transitions in social roles, relationships, and identity, which can further impact older adults' sense of self-worth, purpose, and fulfillment.

Understanding the needs of aging parents requires a holistic and person-centered approach that takes into account their individual preferences, values, and goals. Each aging parent has unique strengths, vulnerabilities, and preferences, shaped by factors such as genetics, lifestyle, personal history, and cultural background. By taking the time to understand their parents' needs and preferences, caregivers can provide more personalized and effective care that promotes their parents' health, well-being, and dignity.

The Importance of Compassionate Care

Compassionate care is a fundamental aspect of caregiving that emphasizes empathy, kindness, and respect for the inherent dignity and worth of every individual. When it comes to caring for aging parents, compassion is essential for fostering trust, building rapport, and creating a supportive and nurturing environment that honors their autonomy and independence. Compassionate care goes beyond meeting the physical needs of aging parents—it involves listening to their concerns, validating their emotions, and empowering them to make decisions about their care and well-being.

There are several reasons why compassionate care is important for aging parents:

1. Preserving dignity and respect: Aging can be a time of vulnerability and dependency, as older adults may experience declines in physical health, cognitive function, and independence. Providing compassionate care allows caregivers to honor their parents' dignity and respect their autonomy, even in the face of challenges and limitations. By treating aging parents with empathy, kindness, and respect, caregivers help preserve their sense of self-worth, promoting their overall well-being and quality of life.

2. Fostering emotional connection and support: Compassionate care involves fostering emotional connection and support between caregivers and aging parents, creating a safe and nurturing environment where older adults feel valued, heard, and understood. By expressing empathy, compassion, and understanding, caregivers help alleviate feelings of loneliness, anxiety, and sadness in their aging parents, promoting emotional well-being and resilience.

3. Enhancing quality of life: Compassionate care enhances the quality of life for aging parents by addressing their physical, emotional, and social needs in a holistic and person-centered manner. By providing personalized and meaningful support, caregivers help older adults maintain their independence,

autonomy, and sense of purpose, enabling them to live life to the fullest despite the challenges of aging.

4. Promoting health and well-being: Compassionate care promotes the health and well-being of aging parents by addressing their physical, emotional, and social needs in a proactive and preventive manner. By providing support with activities of daily living, medication management, and healthcare coordination, caregivers help older adults maintain their physical health and independence, reducing the risk of falls, hospitalizations, and other adverse health outcomes.

Practical Strategies for Providing Compassionate Care

Providing compassionate care for aging parents requires intention, empathy, and dedication. Here are some practical strategies for cultivating compassion and providing high-quality care for aging parents:

1. Show empathy and understanding: Empathy is a key component of compassionate care, as it allows caregivers to connect with their aging parents on an emotional level and understand their experiences, feelings, and concerns. Caregivers can show empathy towards their aging parents by acknowledging their emotions, validating their feelings, and offering comfort and support during difficult times.

2. Foster open communication: Open communication is essential for building trust, promoting understanding, and fostering collaboration between caregivers and aging parents. Caregivers can

foster open communication by creating a supportive and nonjudgmental environment where their parents feel comfortable expressing themselves and sharing their thoughts, feelings, and concerns.

3. Respect their autonomy and independence: Respecting the autonomy and independence of aging parents is essential for promoting their dignity, self-worth, and well-being. Caregivers can empower their parents to make decisions about their care and well-being by involving them in the decision-making process, respecting their preferences and choices, and honoring their right to privacy and self-determination.

4. Provide personalized and meaningful support: Providing personalized and meaningful support involves tailoring care and assistance to meet the individual needs, preferences, and goals of aging parents. Caregivers can provide support with activities of daily living, medication management, and healthcare coordination, while also encouraging their parents to engage in activities that bring them joy, fulfillment, and meaning.

5. Take care of yourself: Finally, caregivers must remember to take care of themselves and prioritize their own health and well-being. Providing compassionate care for aging parents can be emotionally and physically demanding, and caregivers may experience stress, burnout, and exhaustion if they neglect their own needs. Caregivers can practice self-care by setting boundaries, seeking support from friends and family members, and accessing respite care services when needed.

Compassionate care is essential for promoting the health, well-being, and dignity of aging parents. By cultivating empathy, kindness, and respect, caregivers can create a supportive and nurturing environment that honors their parents' autonomy, independence, and self-worth.

Compassionate care goes beyond meeting the physical needs of aging parents—it involves enhancing their overall quality of life. By providing compassionate care for aging parents with love, understanding, and dignity, caregivers can create meaningful and fulfilling relationships that enrich the lives of both the parents and their caregivers.

2.3 Overcoming Barriers to Compassion

Caring for aging parents is a significant responsibility that often requires compassion, empathy, and understanding. However, despite caregivers' best intentions, there can be barriers that hinder their ability to provide compassionate care to their aging parents. These barriers may arise from various sources, including personal beliefs and attitudes, societal expectations, and practical challenges. By understanding and addressing these barriers, caregivers can enhance their ability to provide high-quality care that promotes their aging parents' well-being.

Understanding the Barriers to Compassion

1. Personal Beliefs and Attitudes: One of the primary barriers to compassion for aging parents can stem from caregivers' personal beliefs and attitudes towards aging, illness, and dependency. Negative stereotypes and misconceptions about aging, such as associating old age with decline, weakness, and worthlessness, can lead caregivers to view their aging parents through a lens of pity or disdain rather than empathy and understanding. Similarly, cultural norms and societal expectations around caregiving and filial piety may influence caregivers' attitudes towards their aging parents, shaping their perceptions of their roles and responsibilities.

2. Emotional Distress and Burnout: Caregiving for aging parents can be emotionally and physically demanding, leading to stress, burnout, and compassion fatigue among caregivers. The constant demands of caregiving, coupled with feelings of guilt, frustration, and helplessness, can erode caregivers' capacity for empathy and compassion, making it difficult for them to connect with their aging parents on an emotional level. Additionally, caregivers may experience feelings of resentment or anger towards their aging parents, particularly if they perceive their caregiving responsibilities as burdensome or unfair.

3. Practical Challenges and Constraints: In addition to emotional barriers, caregivers may also face practical challenges and constraints that impede their ability to provide compassionate care to their aging parents. These challenges may include limited time, resources, and support services, as well as competing demands from work, family, and personal life. Caregivers may feel overwhelmed

and stretched thin by the demands of caregiving, making it difficult for them to prioritize their aging parents' needs and well-being.

Strategies for Overcoming Barriers to Compassion

1. Cultivate Self-Compassion: Before caregivers can effectively care for their aging parents with compassion, they must first cultivate self-compassion and kindness towards themselves. This involves acknowledging their own limitations and vulnerabilities as caregivers, and treating themselves with the same empathy and understanding that they extend to others. Caregivers can practice self-compassion by engaging in self-care activities, setting realistic expectations for themselves, and seeking support from friends, family members, or support groups.

2. Challenge Negative Beliefs and Stereotypes: Caregivers can overcome barriers to compassion by challenging negative beliefs and stereotypes about aging and dependency. This may involve educating themselves about the realities of aging, seeking out positive representations of older adults in media and literature, and reframing their perceptions of aging as a natural and normal part of the human experience. By challenging negative beliefs and stereotypes, caregivers can cultivate a more empathetic and compassionate attitude towards their aging parents.

3. Practice Mindfulness and Presence: Mindfulness involves cultivating awareness and acceptance of the present moment, without judgment or attachment. Caregivers can practice mindfulness in their interactions with their aging parents by bringing their full attention and presence to the moment, without getting

caught up in worries or distractions. By practicing mindfulness, caregivers can deepen their connection with their aging parents, enhance their capacity for empathy and understanding, and respond to their parents' needs with compassion and kindness.

4. Seek Support and Guidance: Caregivers can overcome barriers to compassion by seeking support and guidance from others who have experience in caring for aging parents. This may involve reaching out to friends, family members, or support groups for emotional support and practical advice, as well as consulting with healthcare professionals or social workers for guidance on caregiving strategies and resources. By seeking support and guidance, caregivers can gain new perspectives, learn effective coping strategies, and feel less isolated in their caregiving journey.

5. Set Boundaries and Prioritize Self-Care: Setting boundaries and prioritizing self-care is essential for caregivers to maintain their emotional well-being and capacity for compassion. Caregivers can set boundaries by establishing clear limits on their caregiving responsibilities, communicating their needs and limitations to their aging parents and other family members, and seeking help when needed. Additionally, caregivers can prioritize self-care by engaging in activities that nourish their body, mind, and spirit, such as exercise, meditation, praying, hobbies, and socializing with friends.

Caring for aging parents is a profound and complex responsibility that requires compassion, empathy, and understanding. However, caregivers may face barriers to compassion stemming from personal beliefs and attitudes, emotional distress and burnout, and practical challenges and constraints. By cultivating self-compassion, challenging negative beliefs and stereotypes, practicing mindfulness and presence, seeking support and guidance, and setting boundaries and prioritizing self-care, caregivers can overcome these barriers and enhance their ability to provide compassionate care to their aging parents. In doing so, caregivers can create a supportive and nurturing environment that honors their parents' dignity, autonomy, and well-being, and promotes a deeper connection and understanding between generations.

2.4 Cultivating Patience and Understanding

As individuals age, they often encounter a myriad of challenges, ranging from declining physical health and cognitive function to changes in social roles and relationships. For adult children, navigating these challenges alongside their aging parents requires a deep well of patience and understanding. Cultivating patience and understanding is essential for fostering strong, supportive relationships with aging parents, promoting their well-being, and navigating the complexities of aging together.

Cultivating patience and understanding in caregiving relationships with aging parents requires intention, empathy, and commitment. Here are some strategies for nurturing patience and understanding:

1. Be Mindful of Nonverbal Cues: Nonverbal communication, such as facial expressions, body language, and tone of voice, can convey a wealth of information about a person's thoughts, feelings, and

intentions. Caregivers should be mindful of their own nonverbal cues when interacting with their aging parents, as well as attuned to their parents' nonverbal cues to better understand their emotions and needs.

2. Practice Patience and Flexibility: Patience is a virtue, especially when caring for aging parents who may have complex needs and challenges. Caregivers should practice patience and flexibility in their interactions with their aging parents, recognizing that aging is a gradual and ongoing process that requires time, understanding, and adaptability.

3. Set Realistic Expectations: Setting realistic expectations is essential for maintaining patience and understanding in caregiving relationships with aging parents. Caregivers should recognize their own limitations and the limitations of their aging parents, and set realistic goals and expectations for what can be achieved.

4. Seek Support and Respite: Caregiving for aging parents can be emotionally and physically demanding, and caregivers may experience burnout and compassion fatigue if they neglect their own needs. Caregivers should seek support from friends, family members, or support groups, and take regular breaks to recharge and rejuvenate.

Cultivating patience and understanding in caregiving relationships with aging parents is essential for promoting their well-being, fostering strong, supportive relationships, and navigating the complexities of aging together. By practicing active listening, showing empathy and validation, being mindful of nonverbal cues, practicing patience and flexibility, setting realistic expectations, seeking support and respite, and practicing self-care, caregivers can nurture patience and understanding in their interactions with their aging parents. In doing so, caregivers can create a supportive and nurturing environment that honors their parents' dignity, autonomy, and well-being, and promotes a deeper connection and understanding between generations.

Chapter 3: Essential Caregiving Skills

3.1 Communication Strategies for Effective Caregiving

Effective communication is a cornerstone of caregiving for aging parents, facilitating understanding, empathy, and collaboration between caregivers and their loved ones. As aging parents navigate the challenges of aging, including declining physical health, changes in cognitive function, and shifts in social roles and relationships, effective communication becomes even more crucial for meeting their needs and promoting their well-being. By mastering these communication strategies, caregivers can enhance their ability to provide high-quality care that honors their parents' dignity, autonomy, and well-being.

Effective communication is essential for building trust, fostering empathy, and promoting mutual understanding between caregivers and aging parents. Communication serves as a vehicle for expressing needs, preferences, and concerns, as well as for providing information, support, and guidance. In the context of caregiving for aging parents, effective communication plays a crucial role in:

1. Building Strong Relationships: Communication fosters connection and rapport between caregivers and aging parents, creating a supportive and nurturing environment where both parties feel valued, heard, and understood. Strong relationships built on open and honest communication are essential for promoting trust, cooperation, and collaboration in caregiving.

2. Promoting Empathy and Understanding: Effective communication allows caregivers to empathize with their aging parents' experiences, feelings, and concerns, fostering a deeper understanding of their needs and preferences. By listening actively, validating emotions, and offering support and encouragement, caregivers can demonstrate empathy and understanding towards their aging parents, promoting their emotional well-being and resilience.

3. Facilitating Decision-Making and Problem-Solving: Communication is essential for engaging aging parents in decision-making and problem-solving related to their care and well-being. By involving their parents in discussions about care preferences, treatment options, and future planning, caregivers empower them to make informed decisions about their own lives, promoting autonomy and self-determination.

4. Providing Information and Education: Effective communication allows caregivers to provide aging parents with accurate information, education, and resources related to their health, safety, and well-being. By sharing information about medical conditions, treatment options, and available support services, caregivers empower their parents to take an active role in managing their health and making informed decisions about their care.

Essential Communication Skills for Caregiving

1. Active Listening: Active listening entails dedicating full attention to and comprehending what the other individual is expressing, refraining from interruptions or judgments. When interacting with

elderly parents, caregivers can employ active listening by offering undivided attention, sustaining eye contact, and rephrasing their parents' statements to exhibit comprehension and empathy.

2. Empathy and Validation: Empathy is the ability to understand and share the feelings of another person, while validation involves acknowledging and accepting the legitimacy of their emotions. Caregivers can show empathy towards their aging parents by acknowledging their emotions, validating their feelings, and offering comfort and support during difficult times.

3. Clear and Concise Communication: Clear and concise communication is essential for ensuring that messages are understood and acted upon effectively. Caregivers should use simple language, avoid jargon or medical terminology, and provide information in a clear and organized manner.

4. Respectful and Patient Communication: Respectful and patient communication is essential for maintaining dignity, autonomy, and well-being in caregiving relationships. Caregivers should communicate with their aging parents in a respectful and nonjudgmental manner, honoring their preferences, choices, and boundaries.

5. Nonverbal Communication: Nonverbal communication, such as facial expressions, body language, and tone of voice, conveys important information about a person's thoughts, feelings, and intentions. Caregivers should be mindful of their own nonverbal cues when communicating with their aging parents, as well as

attuned to their parents' nonverbal cues to better understand their emotions and needs.

6. Open and Honest Communication: Open and honest communication is essential for building trust and fostering collaboration in caregiving relationships. Caregivers should encourage their aging parents to express themselves openly and honestly, and should respond to their concerns and questions with transparency and honesty.

7. Conflict Resolution Skills: Conflict is a natural and inevitable part of caregiving relationships, but effective communication skills can help caregivers navigate conflicts and disagreements constructively. Caregivers should practice active listening, empathy, and problem-solving skills when resolving conflicts with their aging parents, and should strive to find mutually acceptable solutions that honor their parents' needs and preferences.

Practical Communication Strategies for Caregiving

1. Schedule Regular Check-Ins: Regular check-ins provide opportunities for caregivers and aging parents to communicate openly and address any concerns or questions that may arise. Caregivers can schedule regular check-ins with their parents to discuss their health, well-being, and care preferences, and to provide updates on any changes or developments in their care plan.

2. Use Visual Aids and Written Materials: Visual aids and written materials can help clarify complex information and reinforce key messages for aging parents. Caregivers can use visual aids such as

diagrams, charts, and videos to explain medical conditions, treatment options, and self-care techniques, and can provide written materials such as pamphlets, handouts, and checklists for reference.

3. Encourage Questions and Feedback: Caregivers should encourage their aging parents to ask questions and provide feedback about their care and well-being. By creating a safe and supportive environment where questions and concerns are welcomed, caregivers empower their parents to take an active role in managing their health and advocating for their needs.

4. Be Flexible and Adaptive: Effective communication requires flexibility and adaptability to accommodate the changing needs and preferences of aging parents. Caregivers should be willing to adjust their communication style and approach based on their parents' abilities, preferences, and comfort level, and should be open to feedback and suggestions for improvement.

5. Seek Support and Guidance: Caregivers can seek support and guidance from healthcare professionals, social workers, or support groups to enhance their communication skills and address any challenges or concerns that may arise. By accessing resources and expertise, caregivers can gain new insights and perspectives on effective communication strategies for caregiving.

Effective communication is essential for providing high-quality care to aging parents, fostering understanding, empathy, and collaboration in caregiving relationships. By mastering essential communication skills such as active listening, empathy, clear and concise communication, respectful and patient communication, nonverbal communication, open and honest communication, and conflict resolution skills, caregivers can enhance their ability to meet their parents' needs and promote their well-being. Practical communication strategies such as scheduling regular check-ins, using visual aids and written materials, encouraging questions and feedback, being flexible and adaptive, and seeking support and guidance can further support effective communication in caregiving relationships. By prioritizing effective communication, caregivers can create a supportive and nurturing environment that honors their parents' dignity, autonomy, and well-being, and promotes a deeper connection and understanding between generations.

3.2 Practical Tips for Assisting with Daily Activities

Assisting aging parents with daily activities is a fundamental aspect of caregiving that requires empathy, patience, and practical skills. As individuals age, they may experience changes in physical health, cognitive function, and mobility that impact their ability to perform activities of daily living independently. Caregivers play a crucial role in supporting their aging parents with these tasks, helping to maintain their independence, dignity, and quality of life. By mastering these skills, caregivers can enhance their ability to provide high-quality care that meets their parents' needs and preferences.

Assisting aging parents with daily activities is essential for promoting their well-being, safety, and independence. Daily activities, also known as activities of daily living (ADLs) and instrumental activities of daily living (IADLs), encompass a range of tasks that individuals perform on a regular basis to meet their basic needs and maintain their independence. Some common ADLs include:

1. Personal Care: Personal care activities include tasks such as bathing, grooming, dressing, toileting, and oral hygiene. These activities are essential for maintaining personal hygiene, physical health, and well-being.

2. Mobility: Mobility activities include tasks such as walking, transferring from bed to chair, and using mobility aids such as walkers or wheelchairs. Maintaining mobility is crucial for independence and quality of life, as it allows individuals to engage in daily activities and social interactions.

3. Eating and Nutrition: Eating and nutrition activities include tasks such as meal preparation, feeding, and assistance with eating. Proper nutrition is essential for maintaining overall health and well-being, particularly in older adults who may have specific dietary needs or restrictions.

4. Medication Management: Medication management activities include tasks such as medication administration, medication reminders, and organizing medications. Proper medication management is essential for managing chronic conditions, preventing adverse drug interactions, and promoting medication adherence.

5. Household Tasks: Household tasks include tasks such as cleaning, laundry, shopping, and managing finances. These activities are important for maintaining a safe and comfortable living environment, as well as for promoting independence and autonomy.

Practical Tips for Assisting with Daily Activities

1. Personal Care:

> a. Establish a Routine: Establishing a consistent daily routine can help aging parents feel more comfortable and confident in their personal care routines. Caregivers can create a schedule for bathing, grooming, and dressing that aligns with their parents' preferences and abilities.

> b. Provide Assistance as Needed: Offer assistance with personal care tasks such as bathing, grooming, and dressing, while respecting your parents' privacy and dignity. Provide verbal cues and physical support as needed, and allow your parents to participate in the process as much as possible.

> c. Adapt the Environment: Make adjustments to the bathroom and bedroom environment to enhance safety and accessibility for aging parents. Install grab bars, non-slip mats, and shower benches in the bathroom, and ensure that clothing and personal care items are within easy reach.

2. Mobility:

a. Encourage Physical Activity: Encourage aging parents to engage in regular physical activity to maintain strength, flexibility, and mobility. Offer support and encouragement for activities such as walking, chair exercises, and gentle stretching exercises.

b. Assist with Transfers: Provide assistance with transferring from bed to chair, chair to toilet, and chair to standing position as needed. Use proper body mechanics and assistive devices such as transfer belts or gait belts to ensure safety and prevent falls.

c. Use Mobility Aids: If aging parents use mobility aids such as walkers, canes, or wheelchairs, ensure that these devices are properly fitted and in good working condition. Provide assistance with using mobility aids safely and confidently, and encourage regular maintenance and adjustments as needed.

3. Eating and Nutrition:

a. Prepare Nutritious Meals: Prepare and serve nutritious meals that meet your aging parents' dietary needs and preferences. Offer a variety of foods from different food groups, and encourage balanced meals that include fruits, vegetables, whole grains, lean proteins, and healthy fats.

b. Assist with Feeding: Provide assistance with feeding if aging parents have difficulty with chewing, swallowing, or self-feeding. Offer small, manageable bites of food, and encourage slow, deliberate chewing and swallowing.

c. Monitor Fluid Intake: Monitor your aging parents' fluid intake and encourage them to drink plenty of water throughout the day. Offer beverages such as herbal tea, or low-sugar juices, and provide reminders to drink fluids regularly.

4. Medication Management:

a. Create a Medication Schedule: Create a medication schedule that outlines the names of medications, dosages, and administration times. Use a pill organizer or medication reminder system to help aging parents keep track of their medications and adhere to their prescribed regimen.

b. Assist with Medication Administration: Provide assistance with medication administration as needed, ensuring that aging parents take the correct medications in the right doses and at the prescribed times. Use techniques such as pill splitting, crushing, or mixing with food or liquid if necessary.

c. Communicate with Healthcare Providers: Keep lines of communication open with your aging parents' healthcare providers, including doctors, pharmacists, and nurses. Share information about medication changes, side effects, and concerns, and seek guidance and advice as needed.

5. Household Tasks:

a. Delegate Tasks: Delegate household tasks among family members or enlist the help of professional caregivers or home care aides to assist with cleaning, laundry, shopping, and other household chores. Create a schedule or chore chart to ensure that tasks are completed regularly and efficiently.

b. Simplify Tasks: Simplify household tasks by breaking them down into smaller, manageable steps and using adaptive equipment or assistive devices as needed. Focus on essential tasks that promote safety and comfort, and prioritize tasks based on urgency and importance.

c. Plan and Organize: Plan and organize household tasks in advance to streamline the process and reduce stress and anxiety. Create a weekly or monthly calendar that outlines cleaning, shopping, and other tasks, and allocate time for rest and relaxation.

Assisting aging parents with daily activities is a multifaceted and essential aspect of caregiving that requires empathy, patience, and practical skills. By mastering practical tips for assisting with personal care, mobility, eating and nutrition, medication management, and household tasks, caregivers can enhance their ability to meet their parents' needs and promote their well-being and independence. Through delivering empathetic and proficient care that respects the dignity, autonomy, and preferences of their parents, caregivers can foster a nurturing and supportive atmosphere that enhances the well-being of both themselves and their elderly parents.

3.3 Managing Medications and Healthcare Needs

As individuals age, they often require assistance with managing medications and healthcare needs due to changes in health status, cognitive function, and mobility. Caregivers play a critical role in ensuring that aging parents receive safe and effective medical care, including medication management, healthcare coordination, and advocacy. Managing medications and healthcare needs requires caregivers to possess essential skills such as organization, communication, and attention to detail, as well as empathy, patience, and compassion. By mastering these skills, caregivers can enhance their ability to provide high-quality care that promotes their parents' health, well-being, and independence.

Managing medications and healthcare needs is essential for promoting the health, safety, and quality of life of aging parents. As individuals age, they may experience multiple chronic conditions, complex medication regimens, and frequent interactions with healthcare providers. Effective management of medications and healthcare needs is crucial for:

1. Medication Safety: Proper medication management helps prevent medication errors, adverse drug interactions, and medication-related complications. Aging parents may be at

increased risk of medication errors due to factors such as memory loss, vision changes, and difficulty with medication administration.

2. Health Maintenance: Regular monitoring and management of chronic conditions, preventive screenings, and vaccinations are essential for maintaining optimal health and well-being in aging parents. Caregivers play a key role in facilitating access to healthcare services, scheduling appointments, and advocating for appropriate medical care.

3. Treatment Adherence: Adherence to prescribed medication regimens and treatment plans is critical for managing chronic conditions, preventing disease progression, and optimizing health outcomes. Caregivers can support their aging parents with medication adherence through reminders, organization, and assistance with medication administration.

4. Healthcare Coordination: Coordinating healthcare services and communicating with healthcare providers is essential for ensuring continuity of care and addressing the evolving needs of aging parents. Caregivers serve as advocates for their parents in healthcare settings, providing information, asking questions, and advocating for their parents' preferences and concerns.

Practical Strategies for Managing Medications and Healthcare Needs

1. Organize Medications:

a. Create a Medication List: Compile a comprehensive list of all medications that aging parents are taking, including prescription medications, over-the-counter medications, vitamins, and supplements. Include information such as the name of the medication, dosage, frequency, and purpose.

b. Use a Pill Organizer: Use a pill organizer or medication dispenser to organize medications by day and time, making it easier for aging parents to keep track of their medication schedule. Choose a pill organizer with compartments labeled with the days of the week and times of day to facilitate medication adherence.

c. Set Up a Medication Reminder System: Establish a medication reminder system to alert aging parents when it is time to take their medications. Use techniques such as alarms on a smartphone or clock, written reminders placed in visible locations, or medication reminder apps to prompt medication administration.

2. Communicate with Healthcare Providers:

a. Maintain Open Communication: Keep lines of communication open with healthcare providers, including doctors, pharmacists, and nurses. Share information about aging parents' medical history, current medications, and treatment plans, and ask questions or voice concerns about medications or healthcare recommendations.

b. Attend Medical Appointments: Accompany aging parents to medical appointments to provide support, gather information, and ensure that healthcare providers have a complete understanding of their health status and needs. Take notes during appointments and ask questions to clarify information or address concerns.

c. Advocate for Healthcare Needs: Advocate for aging parents' healthcare needs and preferences by communicating their wishes, concerns, and treatment goals to healthcare providers. Be proactive in seeking appropriate medical care, referrals to specialists, and follow-up appointments as needed.

3. Monitor Medication Adherence:

a. Observe Medication Taking: Observe aging parents as they take their medications to ensure that they are taking the correct medications in the right doses and at the prescribed times. Offer assistance with medication administration if needed, using techniques such as opening medication bottles.

b. Address Barriers to Adherence: Identify and address any barriers to medication adherence that aging parents may be experiencing, such as forgetfulness, confusion, or side effects. Work together to develop strategies for overcoming these barriers, such as setting up reminders, using pill organizers, or adjusting medication schedules.

c. Encourage Open Communication: Encourage aging parents to communicate openly about their experiences with medications, including any side effects, concerns, or changes in symptoms. Be supportive and nonjudgmental in your response, and work together to find solutions that address their needs and preferences.

4. Coordinate Healthcare Services:

a. Keep Medical Records Organized: Keep aging parents' medical records organized and easily accessible, including copies of medical history, test results, and treatment plans. Use a designated folder or binder to store documents, and make copies for reference during medical appointments or emergencies.

b. Facilitate Communication Between Providers: Facilitate communication between healthcare providers by sharing relevant information and updates about aging parents' health status, treatments, and medications. Use a communication log or electronic health record system to track interactions and ensure continuity of care.

c. Advocate for Comprehensive Care: Advocate for comprehensive care that addresses all aspects of aging parents' health and well-being, including physical, emotional, and social needs. Work with healthcare providers to develop personalized care plans that consider aging parents' preferences, goals, and values.

Managing medications and healthcare needs for aging parents requires caregivers to possess essential skills such as organization, communication, and attention to detail, as well as empathy, patience, and compassion. By implementing practical strategies such as organizing medications, communicating with healthcare providers, monitoring medication adherence, and coordinating healthcare services, caregivers can enhance their ability to provide high-quality care that promotes their parents' health, well-being, and independence. By serving as advocates for their aging parents in healthcare settings and ensuring access to safe and effective medical care, caregivers play a crucial role in supporting their parents' journey through aging with dignity and respect.

3.4 Creating a Safe and Comfortable Environment

Creating a safe and comfortable environment is a crucial aspect of caregiving for aging parents. As individuals age, they may experience changes in physical health, mobility, and sensory function that affect their ability to navigate and interact with their surroundings. Caregivers play a vital role in ensuring that aging parents have a supportive environment that promotes their safety, well-being, and independence. By mastering these skills, caregivers can enhance their ability to provide high-quality care that meets their parents' needs and preferences.

Creating a safe and comfortable environment is essential for promoting the health, safety, and well-being of aging parents. As individuals age, they may be more susceptible to accidents, falls, and injuries due to factors such as decreased mobility, impaired vision, and cognitive changes. Additionally, aging parents may experience physical discomfort or sensory sensitivities that impact their comfort and quality of life. Creating a safe and comfortable environment is important for:

1. Preventing Accidents and Injuries: A safe environment reduces the risk of accidents, falls, and injuries that can have serious consequences for aging parents' health and independence. Simple modifications and precautions can minimize hazards and promote safety in the home environment.

2. Supporting Independence and Autonomy: A comfortable environment fosters independence and autonomy by enabling aging parents to navigate their surroundings confidently and perform activities of daily living with ease. Accessible and user-friendly design features promote autonomy and empower aging parents to maintain control over their daily routines.

3. Enhancing Quality of Life: A comfortable environment enhances quality of life by promoting physical comfort, emotional well-being, and social engagement. By creating a nurturing and inviting atmosphere, caregivers can cultivate a sense of belonging and security that contributes to overall happiness and satisfaction.

4. Facilitating Aging in Place: Creating a safe and comfortable environment allows aging parents to age in place safely and

comfortably, avoiding the need for institutional care or relocation to assisted living facilities. Aging in place promotes continuity of care, familiarity, and independence, while preserving dignity and autonomy.

Practical Strategies for Creating a Safe and Comfortable Environment

1. Assess the Home Environment:

a. Conduct a Safety Assessment: Evaluate the home environment for potential hazards and safety risks, such as uneven flooring, loose rugs, cluttered pathways, and inadequate lighting. Identify areas that require modification or improvement to enhance safety and accessibility for aging parents.

b. Consider Universal Design Principles: Apply universal design principles to create a home environment that is accessible and user-friendly for individuals of all ages and abilities. Incorporate features such as wide doorways, grab bars, lever-style door handles, and non-slip flooring to promote safety and convenience.

c. Adapt to Changing Needs: Anticipate changes in aging parents' needs and abilities over time, and adapt the home environment accordingly. Make modifications such as installing stairlifts, ramps, or bathroom grab bars as needed to accommodate evolving mobility challenges and promote independence.

2. Enhance Safety Measures:

a. Install Home Safety Devices: Install home safety devices such as smoke detectors, carbon monoxide detectors, and fire extinguishers to protect against emergencies and hazards. Test and maintain these devices regularly to ensure they are in proper working condition.

b. Secure Medications and Hazardous Substances: Store medications, cleaning supplies, and other hazardous substances out of reach or in locked cabinets to prevent accidental ingestion or misuse. Use childproof locks or safety latches to restrict access to cabinets and drawers containing potentially harmful items.

c. Remove Tripping Hazards: Minimize tripping hazards such as loose rugs, electrical cords, and cluttered pathways by securing or removing these items from high-traffic areas. Use non-slip mats and rugs to prevent slips and falls, particularly in bathrooms and kitchens.

3. Promote Comfort and Accessibility:

a. Optimize Lighting: Ensure adequate lighting throughout the home to promote visibility and reduce the risk of falls and accidents. Use a combination of natural and artificial lighting sources to illuminate key areas such as hallways, staircases, and entryways.

b. Create Comfortable Living Spaces: Create comfortable living spaces that promote relaxation, rest, and socialization for aging parents. Arrange furniture in a functional and ergonomic layout, and incorporate cozy seating areas, soft furnishings, and personal touches to enhance comfort and well-being.

c. Provide Assistive Devices and Equipment: Provide aging parents with assistive devices and equipment such as mobility aids, hearing aids, and adaptive utensils to facilitate daily activities and promote independence. Ensure that these devices are properly fitted, maintained, and used as recommended.

4. Foster Emotional Well-Being:

a. Promote Social Engagement: Encourage aging parents to maintain social connections and engage in meaningful activities that promote socialization and fulfillment. Arrange regular visits with friends and family members, participate in community events, and explore hobbies and interests together.

b. Offer Emotional Support: Offer emotional support and companionship to aging parents by actively listening, empathizing, and validating their feelings and concerns. Create opportunities for open communication and expression of emotions, and provide reassurance and encouragement during times of stress or uncertainty.

c. Respect Privacy and Dignity: Respect aging parents' privacy and dignity by honoring their preferences, boundaries, and personal space. Encourage autonomy and independence in decision-making, and involve aging parents in discussions about their care and living arrangements.

Creating a safe and comfortable environment is a fundamental aspect of caregiving for aging parents that requires caregivers to possess essential skills such as organization, communication, and attention to detail, as well as empathy, patience, and compassion. By implementing practical strategies such as assessing the home environment, enhancing safety measures, promoting comfort and accessibility, and fostering emotional well-being, caregivers can create a supportive and nurturing environment that promotes their parents' health, safety, and independence. By prioritizing the creation of a safe and comfortable environment, caregivers can provide high-quality care that honors their parents' dignity, autonomy, and well-being, and promotes a sense of security, belonging, and fulfillment in their later years.

Chapter 4: Navigating Family Dynamics

4.1 Addressing Family Roles and Responsibilities

Caring for aging parents is a complex and multifaceted responsibility that often involves navigating family dynamics, roles, and responsibilities. As parents age and require increasing support and care, family members are called upon to come together, collaborate, and make decisions about their parents' well-being and quality of life. However, differing perspectives, expectations, and communication styles can complicate the caregiving process and lead to conflicts and tensions within the family. By fostering open communication, mutual respect, and collaboration, families can work together to provide the best possible care for their aging parents while preserving family relationships and unity.

Addressing family roles and responsibilities is essential for fostering collaboration, coordination, and support within the family caregiving team. As aging parents' needs evolve, family members may assume various roles and responsibilities based on their skills, availability, and relationship dynamics. Some key reasons why addressing family roles and responsibilities is important in caring for aging parents include:

1. Shared Decision-Making: Involving family members in decision-making processes ensures that diverse perspectives, preferences, and priorities are considered when planning and implementing care for aging parents. Shared decision-making promotes transparency, consensus-building, and accountability among family members.

2. Equitable Distribution of Care: Clarifying roles and responsibilities helps distribute caregiving tasks and responsibilities among family members in a fair and equitable manner. By identifying each family member's strengths, limitations, and contributions, caregivers can prevent burnout, resentment, and imbalance in caregiving duties.

3. Effective Communication: Clearly defined roles and responsibilities facilitate effective communication and coordination among family members, reducing misunderstandings, conflicts, and tensions. Open communication channels enable family members to express their needs, concerns, and preferences openly and collaboratively.

4. Respect for Individual Boundaries: Recognizing and respecting individual boundaries and limitations promotes autonomy, self-care, and well-being among family caregivers. Respecting each family member's unique needs, preferences, and capacities fosters a supportive and inclusive caregiving environment.

Strategies for Addressing Family Roles and Responsibilities

1. Initiate Open and Honest Discussions:

> a. Schedule Family Meetings: Schedule regular family meetings to discuss aging parents' care needs, preferences, and goals openly and collaboratively. Set an agenda, establish ground rules for communication, and provide opportunities for all family members to participate and contribute to the discussion.

b. Foster an Inclusive Environment: Foster an inclusive environment where all family members feel comfortable expressing their perspectives, concerns, and suggestions without fear of judgment or criticism. Encourage active listening, empathy, and validation to promote mutual understanding and respect.

c. Seek Input from Aging Parents: Involve aging parents in discussions about their care preferences, priorities, and goals to ensure that their voices are heard and respected. Respect their autonomy and decision-making authority, and empower them to participate in decisions about their own care and well-being.

2. Clarify Roles and Responsibilities:

a. Identify Strengths and Skills: Identify each family member's strengths, skills, and capacities, and assign caregiving tasks and responsibilities accordingly. Consider factors such as availability, proximity, and expertise when determining roles within the caregiving team.

b. Delegate Tasks Appropriately: Delegate caregiving tasks and responsibilities based on each family member's preferences, availability, and comfort level. Distribute tasks such as personal care, household chores, financial management, and healthcare coordination among family members to prevent caregiver burnout and overload.

c. Establish Boundaries and Expectations: Establish clear boundaries and expectations for each family member's involvement in caregiving, including roles, responsibilities, and commitments. Communicate openly about expectations regarding communication, decision-making, and participation in caregiving activities.

3. Foster Collaboration and Teamwork:

a. Encourage Collaboration: Encourage collaboration and teamwork among family members by fostering a supportive and cooperative caregiving environment. Emphasize the importance of working together towards common goals and objectives, and recognize and appreciate each family member's contributions to caregiving.

b. Share Information and Resources: Share information, resources, and caregiving tasks among family members to promote transparency, efficiency, and effectiveness in caregiving. Use technology tools such as shared calendars, online document repositories, and group messaging platforms to facilitate communication and collaboration.

c. Seek Outside Support: Seek outside support from professional caregivers, healthcare professionals, and community resources to supplement family caregiving efforts and provide additional support and assistance as needed. Acknowledge when additional help is required and be open to seeking assistance from external sources.

4. Manage Conflict and Resentment:

a. Address Conflict Promptly: Address conflicts, tensions, and disagreements among family members promptly and constructively to prevent escalation and promote resolution. Use active listening, empathy, and problem-solving skills to facilitate dialogue and understanding, and seek common ground and compromise.

b. Foster Forgiveness and Understanding: Foster forgiveness and understanding among family members by acknowledging past grievances, misunderstandings, and hurt feelings. Encourage empathy, compassion, and reconciliation to heal rifts and strengthen family bonds, and focus on moving forward with mutual respect and cooperation.

c. Seek Mediation if Necessary: Seek mediation or professional assistance from family therapists, counselors, or mediators if conflicts persist or escalate despite efforts to resolve them internally. Neutral third parties can help facilitate communication, identify underlying issues, and guide families towards mutually acceptable solutions.

Addressing family roles and responsibilities is essential for fostering collaboration, coordination, and support within the family caregiving team. By initiating open and honest discussions, clarifying roles and responsibilities, fostering collaboration and teamwork, and managing conflict and resentment effectively, families can navigate caregiving responsibilities with greater clarity, cohesion, and unity. By working together to provide the best possible care for their aging parents while preserving family relationships and harmony, families can create a supportive and nurturing caregiving environment that honors their parents' dignity, autonomy, and well-being.

4.2 Resolving Conflicts and Establishing Boundaries

Caring for aging parents is a deeply personal and emotionally charged responsibility that can give rise to conflicts, tensions, and challenges within the family dynamics. As siblings, spouses, and other family members come together to support their aging parents, differing perspectives, expectations, and communication styles may lead to misunderstandings and disagreements. Resolving conflicts and establishing boundaries are essential aspects of navigating family dynamics in caregiving, allowing family members to address issues constructively, protect individual well-being, and maintain healthy relationships. By fostering open communication, empathy, and respect, families can work through conflicts and establish clear boundaries that promote harmony, cooperation, and mutual support.

Resolving conflicts is essential for fostering harmony, understanding, and cooperation within the family caregiving team. Conflicts may arise from differences in caregiving philosophies, decision-making styles, or competing priorities among family members. Failure to address conflicts effectively can lead to resentment, tension, and breakdowns in communication, undermining the caregiving process and negatively impacting the well-being of aging parents. Some key reasons why resolving conflicts is important in caring for aging parents include:

1. Promoting Collaboration: Resolving conflicts facilitates collaboration and teamwork among family members by addressing underlying issues and finding mutually acceptable solutions. Collaboration promotes transparency, accountability, and shared responsibility in caregiving, enhancing the quality and effectiveness of care provided to aging parents.

2. Protecting Relationships: Resolving conflicts helps protect relationships among family members by preventing misunderstandings, resentment, and estrangement. Addressing conflicts with empathy, respect, and understanding fosters mutual respect and appreciation, strengthening bonds and preserving family unity.

3. Improving Communication: Resolving conflicts improves communication among family members by fostering open dialogue, active listening, and honest expression of thoughts and feelings. Effective communication promotes clarity, understanding, and trust, enabling family members to navigate caregiving challenges more effectively and supportively.

4. Enhancing Caregiver Well-Being: Resolving conflicts enhances caregiver well-being by reducing stress, anxiety, and emotional burden associated with unresolved conflicts. Addressing conflicts proactively allows caregivers to set boundaries, prioritize self-care,

and maintain healthy boundaries, preserving their physical and emotional health while providing care for aging parents.

Understanding the Importance of Establishing Boundaries

Establishing boundaries is essential for protecting individual well-being, maintaining balance, and promoting healthy relationships within the family caregiving team. Boundaries define limits, expectations, and acceptable behavior in caregiving relationships, ensuring that each family member's needs, preferences, and autonomy are respected and upheld. Establishing boundaries is important in caring for aging parents for several reasons:

1. Protecting Personal Space: Establishing boundaries protects individual personal space and privacy, allowing family members to maintain autonomy and independence in caregiving relationships. Respecting personal boundaries promotes mutual respect and understanding, reducing conflicts and tension within the family dynamics.

2. Preserving Emotional Health: Establishing boundaries preserves emotional health and well-being by preventing caregiver burnout, exhaustion, and resentment. Setting limits on caregiving responsibilities, expectations, and commitments allows caregivers to prioritize self-care, maintain balance, and prevent caregiver overload.

3. Clarifying Roles and Responsibilities: Establishing boundaries clarifies roles and responsibilities within the caregiving team, preventing misunderstandings and conflicts over caregiving tasks

and decisions. Clearly defined boundaries promote accountability, communication, and collaboration among family members, enhancing the effectiveness and efficiency of caregiving efforts.

4. Promoting Respectful Communication: Establishing boundaries promotes respectful communication and interaction among family members by setting expectations for behavior and communication. Respecting boundaries encourages sensitivity, and consideration in caregiving relationships, fostering a supportive and nurturing caregiving environment.

Strategies for Resolving Conflicts and Establishing Boundaries

1. Practice Active Listening:

> a. Listen with Empathy: Practice active listening by listening with empathy and seeking to understand the underlying emotions and perspectives behind family members' words and actions. Show genuine interest and concern for their feelings and experiences, and validate their emotions with empathy and compassion.

> b. Clarify Understanding: Clarify your understanding of family members' concerns, needs, and perspectives by summarizing their points of view and reflecting back their feelings and emotions. Ask open-ended questions to encourage further exploration and clarification, and avoid making assumptions or judgments.

c. Validate Emotions: Validate family members' emotions and experiences by acknowledging their feelings, concerns, and experiences with empathy and compassion. Express understanding and support for their emotions, even if you may not agree with their perspectives or decisions, and offer reassurance and encouragement.

2. Communicate Effectively:

a. Use "I" Statements: Use "I" statements to express your thoughts, feelings, and concerns assertively and respectfully, focusing on your own experiences rather than attributing blame or criticism to others. Frame your communication in terms of your own observations, feelings, and needs, and avoid making accusatory or confrontational statements.

b. Be Clear and Direct: Be clear and direct in your communication by expressing your thoughts, feelings, and expectations in a straightforward and concise manner. Use clear and specific language to convey your message, and avoid ambiguous or vague communication that may lead to misunderstandings or confusion.

c. Practice Active Problem-Solving: Practice active problem-solving by focusing on finding practical solutions to conflicts and challenges rather than dwelling on past grievances or assigning blame. Collaborate with family members to brainstorm ideas, explore alternatives, and negotiate compromises that address everyone's needs and concerns.

3. Set Clear Boundaries:

a. Identify Your Limits: Identify your personal limits, needs, and priorities in caregiving relationships, and set boundaries accordingly to protect your physical, emotional, and psychological well-being. Be honest with yourself about what you can and cannot reasonably handle, and prioritize self-care and balance in caregiving.

b. Communicate Boundaries Assertively: Communicate your boundaries assertively and respectfully to family members, clearly articulating your needs, preferences, and limitations. Use assertive communication techniques to express your boundaries with confidence and clarity, and avoid apologizing or justifying your boundaries.

c. Enforce Boundaries Consistently: Enforce your boundaries consistently and assertively by setting consequences for boundary violations and sticking to them. Be firm and consistent in upholding your boundaries, and resist pressure or guilt-tripping from family members who may try to challenge or undermine them.

4. Seek Professional Support:

a. Consider Family Therapy: Consider seeking professional support from a family therapist or counselor to facilitate communication, resolve conflicts, and establish healthy boundaries within the family caregiving team. Family therapy provides a neutral and supportive environment for exploring and addressing family dynamics and challenges.

b. Engage in Mediation: Engage in mediation or conflict resolution processes facilitated by trained mediators or conflict resolution specialists to address conflicts and disputes within the family dynamic. Mediation promotes constructive dialogue, negotiation, and resolution of conflicts in a collaborative and respectful manner.

c. Consult with Caregiving Professionals: Consult with caregiving professionals such as social workers, geriatric care managers, or elder law attorneys for guidance and support in navigating family dynamics and caregiving challenges. Caregiving professionals can offer practical advice, resources, and referrals to assist families in addressing conflicts and establishing boundaries effectively.

Resolving conflicts and establishing boundaries are essential aspects of navigating family dynamics in caring for aging parents, allowing family members to address issues constructively, protect individual well-being, and maintain healthy relationships. By practicing active listening, communicating effectively, setting clear boundaries, and seeking professional support when needed, families can navigate conflicts and establish boundaries that promote harmony, cooperation, and mutual support in caregiving relationships. By fostering open communication, empathy, and respect, families can work through conflicts and establish clear boundaries that promote harmony, cooperation, and mutual support. Through collaborative efforts and a commitment to understanding and empathy, families can provide the best possible care for their aging parents while preserving family relationships and unity.

4.3 Building a Support Network

Caring for aging parents is a significant responsibility that often requires the support and collaboration of family members, friends, and community resources. Building a support network is essential for caregivers to navigate the challenges of caregiving, manage stress, and prevent burnout. Additionally, a strong support network provides emotional, practical, and informational support, enhancing caregivers' ability to provide high-quality care for their aging parents. By fostering connections, seeking assistance, and utilizing available resources, caregivers can create a supportive and resilient network that promotes their well-being and the well-being of their aging parents.

Building a support network is crucial for caregivers in caring for aging parents for several reasons:

1. Emotional Support: Caring for aging parents can be emotionally challenging, evoking feelings of stress, guilt, and sadness. A support network provides emotional support by offering empathy, validation, and companionship, helping caregivers cope with the emotional demands of caregiving and reduce feelings of isolation and loneliness.

2. Practical Support: A support network offers practical assistance with caregiving tasks such as transportation, meal preparation, and household chores, alleviating the burden on primary caregivers and promoting balance and self-care. Practical support allows caregivers to focus on providing quality care for their aging parents while addressing their own needs and responsibilities.

3. Informational Support: A support network provides informational support by offering guidance, advice, and resources related to caregiving, aging, and healthcare. Access to reliable information and expertise helps caregivers make informed decisions, navigate complex healthcare systems, and advocate effectively for their aging parents' needs and preferences.

4. Respite Care: A support network enables caregivers to access respite care services such as adult day programs, in-home care, and support groups, providing temporary relief from caregiving responsibilities and preventing caregiver burnout. Respite care allows caregivers to recharge, rest, and attend to their own needs while ensuring continuity of care for their aging parents.

Strategies for Building a Support Network

1. Identify Potential Sources of Support:

> a. Family Members: Identify family members who can provide support and assistance with caregiving tasks, such as siblings, children, and extended family members. Consider each family member's strengths, availability, and willingness

to contribute to caregiving efforts, and discuss expectations and responsibilities openly and collaboratively.

b. Friends and Neighbors: Reach out to friends, neighbors, and acquaintances who may be willing to offer practical assistance, emotional support, or respite care to caregivers. Cultivate relationships with individuals who share common interests, values, or experiences related to caregiving, and explore opportunities for mutual support and collaboration.

c. Community Resources: Research and explore community resources and support services available to caregivers and aging parents, such as senior centers, caregiver support groups, and volunteer organizations. Connect with local agencies, nonprofit organizations, and faith-based groups that offer programs and services tailored to the needs of caregivers and aging adults.

2. Foster Open Communication:

a. Initiate Conversations: Initiate conversations with family members, friends, and community members about caregiving and the challenges and responsibilities involved. Share your experiences, concerns, and needs openly and honestly, and invite others to offer their support, advice, and assistance.

b. Set Realistic Expectations: Set realistic expectations for what types of support and assistance you need from your support network, and communicate these expectations clearly and assertively. Be specific about the types of help you are seeking, whether it be practical assistance, emotional support, or respite care, and express gratitude for any support offered.

c. Be Receptive to Help: Be receptive to offers of help and support from family members, friends, and community resources, even if it means relinquishing some control or accepting assistance with tasks you may prefer to handle yourself. Practice humility and gratitude in receiving support, and reciprocate when possible to maintain a balanced and reciprocal relationship with your support network.

3. Cultivate Connections:

a. Strengthen Family Bonds: Strengthen family bonds and connections by spending quality time together, engaging in shared activities, and fostering open communication and understanding. Cultivate empathy, compassion, and solidarity among family members, and prioritize maintaining positive relationships and connections.

b. Nurture Friendships: Nurture friendships and social connections outside of the caregiving role by staying connected with friends, participating in social activities, and engaging in hobbies and interests that bring joy and fulfillment. Cultivate a diverse network of friendships that provide emotional support, companionship, and perspective outside of the caregiving context.

c. Engage with Community Resources: Engage with community resources and support services that offer opportunities for connection, collaboration, and mutual support among caregivers and aging adults. Participate in caregiver support groups, educational workshops, and community events that provide opportunities for networking, sharing experiences, and accessing resources and information.

4. Utilize Available Resources:

a. Seek Professional Assistance: Seek professional assistance from healthcare providers, social workers, and eldercare professionals who can offer guidance, support, and resources to caregivers and aging parents. Consult with professionals specializing in aging, caregiving, and mental health to address specific challenges and concerns and access appropriate interventions and support services.

b. Access Respite Care Services: Access respite care services such as adult day programs, in-home care, and caregiver support groups that offer temporary relief from caregiving responsibilities and allow caregivers to recharge and attend to their own needs. Utilize respite care services regularly to prevent burnout and maintain balance and well-being.

c. Explore Online Resources: Explore online resources and digital platforms that provide information, support, and community for caregivers and aging adults. Access websites, forums, and social media groups dedicated to caregiving and aging-related topics, where caregivers can connect with peers, share experiences, and access resources and support.

Building a support network is essential for caregivers in caring for aging parents, providing emotional, practical, and informational support that enhances their ability to provide high-quality care while maintaining their own well-being. By identifying potential sources of support, fostering open communication, cultivating connections, and utilizing available resources, caregivers can create a resilient and supportive network that promotes their well-being and the well-being of their aging parents. Through collaboration, compassion, and mutual support, caregivers can navigate the challenges of caregiving with greater resilience, strength, and solidarity, knowing that they are not alone in their caregiving journey.

4.4 Understanding the Impact of Caregiving on Family Relationships

Caring for aging parents can profoundly impact family relationships, dynamics, and roles, as family members come together to provide support, assistance, and care for their loved ones. While caregiving can strengthen bonds and foster unity within the family, it can also give rise to conflicts, tensions, and challenges as caregivers navigate caregiving responsibilities, decision-making, and communication. Understanding the impact of caregiving on family relationships is essential for caregivers to anticipate and address potential challenges, foster resilience, and maintain positive and supportive relationships within the family dynamics. By fostering open communication, empathy, and cooperation, families can navigate caregiving challenges while preserving and strengthening their relationships with one another.

Caring for aging parents can have a profound impact on family relationships in various ways:

1. Shifting Roles and Responsibilities: Caregiving often requires family members to assume new roles and responsibilities within the family dynamic, such as primary caregiver, decision-maker, or financial manager. These role changes can disrupt established family roles and dynamics, leading to conflicts, tensions, and adjustments as family members navigate their evolving roles and responsibilities.

2. Changes in Communication Patterns: Caregiving can affect communication patterns within the family, as caregivers may need to communicate more frequently and assertively about caregiving tasks, schedules, and decisions. Differences in communication styles, expectations, and preferences among family members can lead to misunderstandings, conflicts, and breakdowns in communication, impacting the quality and effectiveness of caregiving relationships.

3. Emotional Stress and Burden: Caregiving can evoke a range of emotions among family members, including stress, anxiety, guilt, and grief, as they navigate the challenges and demands of caregiving. Emotional stress and burden can strain family relationships, leading to resentment, frustration, and tension

among caregivers and other family members who may feel overwhelmed or unsupported in their caregiving roles.

4. Financial Strain and Resources: Caregiving can impose financial strain on families, as caregivers may need to reduce their work hours, take unpaid leave, or incur out-of-pocket expenses to provide care for aging parents. Financial strain can create tension and conflict within the family, particularly if family members disagree on financial decisions or contributions to caregiving expenses, leading to disputes and resentment.

5. Impact on Personal Relationships: Caregiving can impact personal relationships within the family, as caregivers may prioritize caregiving responsibilities over other obligations and commitments, such as work, social activities, or personal interests. Changes in priorities and availability can strain personal relationships, leading to feelings of neglect, isolation, or abandonment among family members who may feel sidelined or marginalized in the caregiving process.

Strategies for Navigating Family Dynamics

1. Foster Open Communication:

    a. Initiate Regular Family Meetings: Initiate regular family meetings to discuss caregiving responsibilities, concerns, and decisions openly and collaboratively. Set an agenda, establish ground rules for communication, and provide opportunities for all family members to share their perspectives, concerns, and suggestions.

b. Practice Active Listening: Practice active listening by listening with empathy and attention to family members' thoughts, feelings, and concerns. Validate their experiences and perspectives with empathy and understanding, and avoid interrupting or dismissing their emotions or opinions.

c. Express Needs and Boundaries: Express your own needs, boundaries, and limitations in caregiving relationships assertively and respectfully. Be honest and transparent about your capacity to provide care and the support you require from other family members, and encourage open dialogue and collaboration in addressing caregiving challenges.

2. Share Caregiving Responsibilities:

a. Distribute Tasks Equitably: Distribute caregiving tasks and responsibilities among family members equitably, taking into account each member's strengths, availability, and preferences. Avoid burdening one family member with the majority of caregiving responsibilities, and foster a sense of shared accountability and collaboration in caregiving efforts.

b. Coordinate Care Plans: Coordinate care plans and schedules collaboratively with family members to ensure continuity of care and support for aging parents. Share information, resources, and updates about caregiving tasks, appointments, and medications, and establish clear channels of communication for sharing relevant information and coordinating care effectively.

c. Seek Outside Assistance: Seek outside assistance from professional caregivers, healthcare providers, or community resources to supplement family caregiving efforts and provide additional support and assistance as needed. Acknowledge when additional help is required and be open to seeking assistance from external sources to lighten the caregiving burden and promote family unity.

3. Foster Empathy and Understanding:

a. Practice Empathy: Practice empathy and understanding in caregiving relationships by acknowledging and validating family members' emotions, experiences, and perspectives. Cultivate empathy by putting yourself in others' shoes and considering their feelings and needs with compassion and sensitivity.

b. Offer Support and Encouragement: Offer support and encouragement to family members who may be struggling with caregiving responsibilities or emotional stress. Express gratitude and appreciation for their efforts and contributions to caregiving, and provide reassurance and encouragement during challenging times.

c. Seek Professional Support: Seek professional support from therapists, counselors, or support groups specializing in caregiving and family dynamics to address conflicts, tensions, or challenges within the family dynamic. Professional support can offer insights, strategies, and interventions to promote empathy, understanding, and resolution of family conflicts and tensions.

4. Maintain Boundaries and Self-Care:

a. Establish Personal Boundaries: Establish clear boundaries around caregiving responsibilities, commitments, and self-care practices to protect your physical, emotional, and psychological well-being. Communicate your boundaries assertively and respectfully to family members, and prioritize self-care activities that promote balance and resilience in caregiving relationships.

b. Practice Self-Care: Prioritize self-care practices such as exercise, relaxation, hobbies, and social activities to recharge and replenish your energy and resilience as a caregiver. Make time for activities that bring you joy and fulfillment, and enlist support from family members or community resources to ensure you have the time and space to care for yourself.

c. Seek Respite and Support: Seek respite care services and support from family members, friends, or community resources to take breaks from caregiving responsibilities and recharge your batteries. Utilize respite care services regularly to prevent burnout and maintain balance and well-being in your caregiving relationships.

Caring for aging parents can have a profound impact on family relationships, dynamics, and well-being, as caregivers navigate the challenges and demands of caregiving while maintaining positive and supportive relationships with their loved ones. By fostering open communication, sharing caregiving responsibilities, practicing empathy and understanding, and maintaining boundaries and self-care practices, families can navigate the complexities of caregiving with resilience, compassion, and unity. Through collaboration, cooperation, and mutual support, families can preserve and strengthen their relationships while providing the best possible care for their aging parents.

Chapter 5: Promoting Emotional Well-being

5.1 Supporting Emotional Health and Resilience

Caring for aging parents is a complex and demanding responsibility that can have significant implications for caregivers' emotional health and well-being. As caregivers navigate the challenges of providing physical, emotional, and logistical support to their aging parents, they may experience a range of emotions, including stress, anxiety, guilt, and grief. Supporting emotional health and resilience is essential for caregivers to cope with the demands of caregiving, manage stress effectively, and maintain a sense of well-being and balance in their lives. By fostering self-awareness, seeking support, and practicing self-care, caregivers can enhance their emotional health and resilience, enabling them to provide compassionate and effective care for their aging parents while preserving their own well-being.

Supporting emotional health and resilience is crucial for caregivers in caring for aging parents for several reasons:

1. Coping with Stress and Burnout: Caregiving can be physically, emotionally, and mentally taxing, leading to stress, burnout, and exhaustion among caregivers. Supporting emotional health and resilience helps caregivers cope with the demands of caregiving, manage stress effectively, and prevent burnout, enabling them to sustain their caregiving efforts over time.

2. Promoting Quality of Care: Caregivers' emotional well-being directly impacts the quality of care they provide to their aging parents. Caregivers who are emotionally healthy and resilient are better able to provide compassionate, patient-centered care, communicate effectively, and maintain positive relationships with their aging parents, enhancing the overall quality of care provided.

3. Preserving Family Relationships: Emotional health and resilience are essential for preserving family relationships and harmony within the caregiving team. Caregivers who are emotionally healthy and resilient are better equipped to navigate conflicts, communicate assertively, and collaborate effectively with other family members, fostering unity and cooperation in caregiving relationships.

4. Enhancing Personal Well-being: Supporting emotional health and resilience is essential for caregivers' personal well-being and quality of life. Caregivers who prioritize their emotional health and well-being are more likely to experience greater satisfaction, fulfillment, and meaning in their caregiving role, as well as improved physical health and overall well-being.

Strategies for Promoting Emotional Well-being

1. Foster Self-awareness:

> a. Acknowledge Emotions: Acknowledge and validate your emotions as a caregiver, including feelings of stress, frustration, sadness, and guilt. Recognize that experiencing a range of emotions is normal and natural in caregiving

relationships, and give yourself permission to feel and express your emotions without judgment or self-criticism.

b. Identify Triggers: Identify triggers and stressors that contribute to negative emotions and feelings of overwhelm in caregiving situations. Reflect on specific situations, tasks, or interactions that evoke strong emotional reactions, and explore strategies for managing and mitigating these triggers effectively.

c. Practice Mindfulness: Practice mindfulness and self-awareness techniques to cultivate present moment awareness and non-judgmental acceptance of your thoughts, feelings, and sensations. Incorporate mindfulness practices such as deep breathing, meditation, or body scan exercises into your daily routine to reduce stress, enhance emotional regulation, and promote self-awareness.

2. Seek Support:

a. Reach Out to Others: Reach out to family members, friends, or support groups for emotional support, validation, and companionship in caregiving. Share your experiences, concerns, and feelings openly and honestly with trusted individuals who can offer empathy, understanding, and encouragement during challenging times.

b. Join a Caregiver Support Group: Join a caregiver support group or online community to connect with other caregivers who are facing similar challenges and experiences.

Participate in group discussions, share resources, and exchange advice and support with fellow caregivers, fostering a sense of solidarity and camaraderie in your caregiving journey.

c. Consult with a Therapist: Consult with a therapist, counselor, or mental health professional for individual counseling or therapy to address specific emotional challenges or concerns related to caregiving. Therapy provides a safe and supportive space to explore your feelings, gain insight into your coping strategies, and develop effective coping skills for managing stress and emotions.

3. Practice Self-care:

a. Prioritize Self-care Activities: Prioritize self-care activities that nourish your physical, emotional, and psychological well-being, such as exercise, relaxation, hobbies, and socializing. Make time for activities that bring you joy, fulfillment, and relaxation, and incorporate self-care practices into your daily routine to replenish your energy and resilience as a caregiver.

b. Set Boundaries: Set boundaries around caregiving responsibilities, commitments, and personal time to protect your emotional health and well-being. Communicate your boundaries assertively and respectfully to family members and other stakeholders involved in caregiving, and prioritize your own needs and self-care practices without guilt or apology.

c. Practice Stress Management: Practice stress management techniques such as deep breathing, progressive muscle relaxation, or guided imagery to reduce stress and promote relaxation in caregiving situations. Experiment with different stress management strategies to find what works best for you, and incorporate them into your daily routine to build resilience and cope with caregiving stressors effectively.

4. Cultivate Resilience:

a. Cultivate Positive Coping Strategies: Cultivate positive coping strategies such as optimism, gratitude, and problem-solving to build resilience and adaptability in caregiving situations. Focus on strengths, successes, and moments of joy in your caregiving journey, and practice gratitude for the meaningful connections and experiences you share with your aging parents.

b. Learn from Challenges: Embrace challenges and setbacks as opportunities for growth, learning, and personal development in caregiving relationships. Reflect on difficult experiences, setbacks, and mistakes as valuable learning opportunities that can strengthen your resilience, enhance your coping skills, and deepen your understanding of yourself and others.

c. Foster Flexibility and Adaptability: Foster flexibility and adaptability in caregiving relationships by remaining open-minded, flexible, and adaptable in the face of changing circumstances and challenges. Embrace uncertainty and ambiguity as natural aspects of caregiving, and approach caregiving with curiosity, creativity, and resilience in navigating unexpected twists and turns in the caregiving journey.

Supporting emotional health and resilience is essential for caregivers in caring for aging parents, enabling them to cope with the demands of caregiving, manage stress effectively, and maintain a sense of well-being and balance in their lives. By fostering self-awareness, seeking support, practicing self-care, and cultivating resilience, caregivers can enhance their emotional health and well-being, enabling them to provide compassionate and effective care for their aging parents while preserving their own well-being. Through self-awareness, self-care, and support from others, caregivers can navigate the challenges of caregiving with greater resilience, strength, and compassion, knowing that they are not alone in their caregiving journey.

5.2 Coping with Grief and Loss

Caring for aging parents can bring about a range of emotions, including joy, fulfillment, and love, but it can also entail experiences of grief and loss as parents age and their health declines. Grief and loss are inherent aspects of the caregiving journey, as caregivers confront changes in their parents' health, independence, and identity, as well as anticipate their eventual passing. Coping with grief and loss is essential for promoting emotional well-being when caring for aging parents, as it allows caregivers to process their emotions, adapt to changes, and find meaning and resilience in their caregiving journey. By acknowledging grief, seeking support, and finding ways to honor and commemorate their parents' lives, caregivers can navigate the complexities of grief and loss with compassion, strength, and healing.

Grief and loss are complex experiences that caregivers may encounter throughout the caregiving journey:

1. Anticipatory Grief: Caregivers often experience anticipatory grief as they anticipate and prepare for their parents' decline in health and eventual passing. Anticipatory grief involves mourning the loss of the parent's physical abilities, cognitive function, independence, and identity, as well as the loss of future plans, dreams, and expectations.

2. Ambiguous Loss: Caregivers may experience ambiguous loss, a type of grief associated with ambiguous or unresolved losses that lack closure or clarity. Ambiguous loss can arise from changes in the parent's health, cognition, or personality, as well as shifts in the caregiving relationship and dynamics, leading to feelings of uncertainty, confusion, and distress.

3. Cumulative Loss: Caregivers may encounter cumulative losses over time as their parents' health declines and caregiving responsibilities increase. Cumulative losses can include the loss of physical abilities, social connections, roles, and routines, as well as the loss of intimacy, companionship, and shared memories with their parents.

4. Secondary Loss: Caregivers may also experience secondary losses associated with caregiving, such as the loss of personal time, freedom, career opportunities, and financial security. Secondary losses can compound the grief and stress experienced by caregivers, leading to feelings of resentment, frustration, and isolation.

Strategies for Coping with Grief and Loss

1. Acknowledge and Validate Emotions:

> a. Recognize Feelings of Grief: Acknowledge and validate your feelings of grief, sadness, and loss as a natural and normal response to the challenges and changes of caregiving. Recognize that experiencing grief does not diminish your love or commitment to your parents, but rather reflects the depth of your connection and attachment to them.

> b. Allow Yourself to Feel: Allow yourself to feel and express your emotions openly and honestly, without judgment or self-criticism. Give yourself permission to grieve in your own way and at your own pace, and honor your emotions as valuable and meaningful expressions of your love and connection to your parents.

> c. Seek Validation and Support: Seek validation and support from family members, friends, or support groups who can offer empathy, understanding, and companionship in your grief journey. Share your feelings, concerns, and experiences openly and honestly with trusted individuals who can

validate and affirm your emotions without judgment or criticism.

2. Practice Self-compassion:

a. Be Kind to Yourself: Be kind and compassionate toward yourself as you navigate the challenges and complexities of caregiving and grief. Practice self-compassion by treating yourself with the same kindness, understanding, and patience you would offer to a loved one experiencing grief and loss.

b. Practice Self-care: Prioritize self-care activities that nourish your physical, emotional, and psychological well-being, such as exercise, relaxation, hobbies, and socializing. Make time for activities that bring you joy, fulfillment, and relaxation, and prioritize your own needs and self-care practices without guilt or apology.

c. Set Realistic Expectations: Set realistic expectations for yourself in caregiving and grief, acknowledging that grief is a natural and ongoing process that unfolds over time. Be gentle with yourself as you navigate the ups and downs of grief, and give yourself permission to take breaks, seek support, and practice self-care as needed.

3. Seek Support:

a. Reach Out to Others: Reach out to family members, friends, or support groups for emotional support, validation, and companionship in your grief journey. Openly and honestly express your experiences, worries, and emotions to trusted individuals who can provide empathy, understanding, and encouragement when facing difficult circumstances.

b. Join a Grief Support Group: Join a grief support group or online community to connect with others who are experiencing similar challenges and emotions related to caregiving and grief. Participate in group discussions, share resources, and exchange advice and support with fellow caregivers, fostering a sense of solidarity and camaraderie in your grief journey.

c. Consult with a Therapist: Consult with a therapist, counselor, or mental health professional for individual counseling or therapy to address specific emotional challenges or concerns related to caregiving and grief. Therapy provides a safe and supportive space to explore your feelings, gain insight into your coping strategies, and develop effective coping skills for managing grief and loss.

4. Honor and Commemorate:

a. Create Rituals and Traditions: Create rituals and traditions to honor and commemorate your parents' lives, memories, and legacies. Establish meaningful rituals or ceremonies that reflect your parents' values, beliefs, and preferences, and incorporate them into your caregiving routine to celebrate their lives and preserve their memory.

b. Share Memories and Stories: Share memories, stories, and anecdotes about your parents with family members, friends, and loved ones to keep their memory alive and honor their legacy. Create opportunities for reminiscing, storytelling, and reflection, and encourage others to share their own memories and experiences as a way of honoring and commemorating your parents' lives.

c. Engage in Meaningful Activities: Engage in meaningful activities and projects that honor your parents' interests, passions, and values, such as volunteering, gardening, or creative pursuits. Dedicate time and energy to activities that bring you joy, fulfillment, and connection with your parents' legacy, and involve family members and loved ones in these activities to foster a sense of shared purpose and connection.

Coping with grief and loss is an essential aspect of promoting emotional well-being when caring for aging parents, as it allows caregivers to process their emotions, adapt to changes, and find meaning and resilience in their caregiving journey. By acknowledging grief, seeking support, practicing self-compassion, and finding ways to honor and commemorate their parents' lives, caregivers can navigate the complexities of grief and loss with compassion, strength, and healing. Through self-awareness, self-care, and support from others, caregivers can find solace and connection in their grief journey, knowing that they are not alone in their experiences of loss and mourning.

5.3 Finding Joy and Meaning in Everyday Moments

Caring for aging parents can be a challenging and demanding responsibility, often accompanied by feelings of stress, sadness, and overwhelm. However, amidst the challenges of caregiving, there are opportunities to find joy and meaning in everyday moments, fostering emotional well-being and resilience. Finding joy and meaning in caregiving involves cultivating gratitude, mindfulness, and resilience, as well as embracing the present moment and cherishing the connections and experiences shared with aging parents. By embracing gratitude, mindfulness, and connection, caregivers can enhance their emotional well-being and find fulfillment and purpose in their caregiving journey.

Finding joy and meaning in everyday moments is essential for promoting emotional well-being when caring for aging parents for several reasons:

1. Enhancing Resilience: Finding joy and meaning in caregiving fosters resilience, enabling caregivers to cope with the challenges and stresses of caregiving more effectively. By focusing on positive aspects of caregiving and cherishing meaningful moments with their aging parents, caregivers can build emotional strength and adaptability in navigating the ups and downs of caregiving.

2. Cultivating Gratitude: Finding joy and meaning involves cultivating gratitude for the blessings, opportunities, and connections present in caregiving relationships. Gratitude helps caregivers shift their focus from difficulties and challenges to

moments of beauty, love, and connection, fostering a sense of appreciation and abundance in their caregiving journey.

3. Embracing Mindfulness: Finding joy and meaning in caregiving involves embracing mindfulness, or present moment awareness, and cherishing the experiences and connections shared with aging parents. Mindfulness allows caregivers to savor the simple pleasures of caregiving, such as moments of laughter, tenderness, and connection, and cultivate a deeper sense of presence and engagement in their caregiving role.

4. Promoting Emotional Well-being: Finding joy and meaning in everyday moments promotes emotional well-being and satisfaction in caregiving relationships. By focusing on positive aspects of caregiving and cherishing meaningful moments with their aging parents, caregivers can experience greater fulfillment, purpose, and satisfaction in their caregiving journey, enhancing their overall well-being and quality of life.

Strategies for Finding Joy and Meaning

1. Cultivate Gratitude:

> a. Practice Gratitude Rituals: Incorporate gratitude rituals into your daily routine, such as keeping a gratitude journal, writing thank-you notes, or reflecting on three things you are grateful for each day. Cultivate an attitude of gratitude by acknowledging and appreciating the blessings, opportunities, and connections present in your caregiving journey.

b. Focus on Silver Linings: Focus on silver linings and positive aspects of caregiving, even amidst challenges and difficulties. Shift your perspective from what is lacking or stressful to what is meaningful, rewarding, and beautiful in your caregiving relationships, and cultivate gratitude for the lessons, growth, and connections fostered through caregiving.

c. Express Appreciation: Express appreciation and gratitude to your aging parents for their love, wisdom, and presence in your life. Take time to acknowledge and thank your parents for the sacrifices they have made and the contributions they have made to your well-being, and express gratitude for the moments of joy, laughter, and connection shared with them.

2. Embrace Mindfulness:

a. Practice Mindful Awareness: Practice mindful awareness by bringing your attention to the present moment and savoring the experiences and connections shared with your aging parents. Engage your senses fully in caregiving activities, such as listening to the sound of your parents' voice, feeling the warmth of their touch, or savoring the taste of a shared meal, and cultivate a sense of presence and appreciation in your interactions.

b. Notice Small Moments of Joy: Notice and appreciate small moments of joy, beauty, and connection in your caregiving relationships. Pay attention to the simple pleasures of caregiving, such as moments of laughter, tenderness, or shared experiences, and cherish these moments as precious gifts that enrich your caregiving journey.

c. Practice Gratitude Walks: Take gratitude walks with your aging parents to appreciate the beauty of nature, the warmth of the sun, and the simple pleasures of being together. Slow down and savor the sights, sounds, and sensations of nature, and cultivate gratitude for the opportunity to share these moments of peace and tranquility with your loved ones.

3. Cherish Connections:

a. Foster Meaningful Conversations: Foster meaningful conversations with your aging parents to deepen your connection and understanding of one another. Take time to listen attentively to your parents' stories, memories, and wisdom, and share your own thoughts, feelings, and experiences openly and honestly, fostering a sense of connection and intimacy in your relationship.

b. Create Shared Experiences: Create opportunities for shared experiences and activities that bring joy, laughter, and connection to your caregiving relationships. Engage in activities that you and your aging parents enjoy together, such as cooking, gardening, or listening to music, and cherish the moments of joy, creativity, and camaraderie shared with one another.

c. Celebrate Milestones and Achievements: Celebrate milestones, achievements, and special occasions with your aging parents to honor their life, accomplishments, and contributions. Take time to commemorate birthdays, anniversaries, and holidays with meaningful rituals, traditions, and celebrations that bring joy, connection, and meaning to your caregiving relationships.

Finding joy and meaning in everyday moments is essential for promoting emotional well-being and resilience when caring for aging parents. By embracing gratitude, mindfulness, and connection, caregivers can enhance their emotional well-being and find fulfillment and purpose in their caregiving journey. Through cultivating gratitude, embracing mindfulness, and cherishing connections with their aging parents, caregivers can experience greater satisfaction, fulfillment, and joy in their caregiving relationships, enriching their lives and the lives of their loved ones. By finding joy and meaning in caregiving, caregivers can navigate the challenges and complexities of caregiving with compassion, strength, and resilience, knowing that every moment shared with their aging parents is a precious gift to be cherished and celebrated.

5.4 Self-care Strategies for Caregivers

Caring for aging parents is a noble and rewarding responsibility, but it can also be emotionally and physically demanding. Caregivers often prioritize the needs of their loved ones above their own, leading to neglect of their own well-being. However, self-care is essential for caregivers to maintain their emotional well-being, prevent burnout, and provide effective care for their aging parents. By prioritizing self-care, caregivers can enhance their resilience, reduce stress, and find balance and fulfillment in their caregiving journey.

Self-care is crucial for caregivers in caring for aging parents for several reasons:

1. Preventing Burnout: Caregiving can be physically, emotionally, and mentally exhausting, leading to burnout and compassion fatigue among caregivers. Self-care helps caregivers recharge their batteries, manage stress effectively, and prevent burnout by prioritizing their own well-being and needs.

2. Enhancing Resilience: Self-care fosters resilience, enabling caregivers to cope with the challenges and stresses of caregiving more effectively. By practicing self-care, caregivers build emotional strength, adaptability, and coping skills, allowing them to navigate the ups and downs of caregiving with greater resilience and grace.

3. Improving Quality of Care: Caregivers' well-being directly impacts the quality of care they provide to their aging parents. Caregivers who prioritize self-care are better able to provide compassionate, patient-centered care, communicate effectively, and maintain positive relationships with their loved ones, enhancing the overall quality of care provided.

4. Promoting Personal Well-being: Self-care is essential for caregivers' personal well-being and quality of life. Caregivers who

prioritize self-care experience greater satisfaction, fulfillment, and meaning in their caregiving role, as well as improved physical health and overall well-being, enabling them to thrive in their caregiving journey.

Strategies for Self-care

1. Prioritize Physical Health:

a. Maintain a Healthy Lifestyle: Maintain a healthy lifestyle by eating nutritious foods, getting regular exercise, and prioritizing adequate sleep. Fuel your body with nourishing foods that provide energy and vitality, engage in physical activities you enjoy, and aim for quality sleep to replenish your energy and resilience as a caregiver.

b. Attend Regular Medical Check-ups: Attend regular medical check-ups with your healthcare provider to monitor your physical health and well-being. Schedule routine screenings, vaccinations, and preventive care appointments to address any health concerns or conditions early and ensure you stay healthy and well in your caregiving role.

c. Practice Relaxation Techniques: Practice relaxation techniques such as deep breathing, meditation, or progressive muscle relaxation to reduce stress and promote relaxation in your body and mind. Incorporate relaxation practices into your daily routine to unwind and recharge, and prioritize activities that bring you peace, joy, and tranquility in your caregiving journey.

2. Nurture Emotional Well-being:

a. Express Emotions: Express your emotions openly and honestly, without judgment or self-criticism. Allow yourself to feel and acknowledge your feelings of stress, sadness, anger, or frustration as a natural and normal response to the challenges and demands of caregiving, and seek support from trusted individuals who can offer empathy and understanding.

b. Engage in Emotional Outlets: Engage in emotional outlets such as journaling, art therapy, or counseling to process your feelings and experiences in caregiving. Find creative ways to express yourself and explore your emotions, thoughts, and concerns in a safe and supportive environment, fostering self-awareness and healing in your caregiving journey.

c. Set Boundaries: Set boundaries around caregiving responsibilities, commitments, and personal time to protect your emotional well-being and prevent burnout. Communicate your boundaries assertively and respectfully to family members and other stakeholders involved in caregiving, and prioritize your own needs and self-care practices without guilt or apology.

3. Cultivate Social Support:

a. Build a Support Network: Build a support network of family members, friends, neighbors, and community resources who can offer practical assistance, emotional support, and companionship in your caregiving journey. Reach out to trusted individuals who can provide encouragement, empathy, and understanding during challenging times, and share your experiences, concerns, and feelings openly and honestly with them.

b. Participate in a Caregiver Support Group: Engage with a caregiver support group or online community where you can connect with others undergoing similar challenges and experiences. Contribute to group conversations, exchange resources, and offer advice and support to fellow caregivers, fostering a bond of solidarity and companionship throughout your caregiving voyage.

c. Seek Professional Support: Seek professional support from therapists, counselors, or support groups specializing in caregiving and caregiver well-being. Consult with a mental health professional for individual counseling or therapy to address specific emotional challenges or concerns related to caregiving, and explore strategies for managing stress, building resilience, and enhancing your emotional well-being.

4. Engage in Meaningful Activities:

a. Pursue Hobbies and Interests: Pursue hobbies, interests, and activities that bring you joy, fulfillment, and relaxation outside of caregiving. Dedicate time and energy to activities you enjoy, whether it's reading, gardening, painting, or playing music, and prioritize self-expression, creativity, and exploration in your life beyond caregiving.

b. Maintain Social Connections: Maintain social connections and relationships with friends, family members, and loved ones outside of caregiving. Make time for socializing, connecting, and sharing experiences with others who bring joy, laughter, and companionship to your life, and nurture meaningful connections that enrich your well-being and sense of belonging.

c. Practice Mindful Activities: Practice mindful activities such as meditation, yoga, or nature walks to cultivate presence, awareness, and gratitude in your daily life. Engage your senses fully in the present moment, savoring the sights, sounds, and sensations of your surroundings, and cultivate a sense of wonder, appreciation, and connection with the world around you.

Self-care is essential for promoting emotional well-being and resilience when caring for aging parents. By prioritizing physical health, nurturing emotional well-being, cultivating social support, and engaging in meaningful activities, caregivers can enhance their resilience, reduce stress, and find balance and fulfillment in their caregiving journey. Through self-awareness, self-care, and support from others, caregivers can navigate the challenges and complexities of caregiving with compassion, strength, and resilience, knowing that taking care of themselves is essential for providing effective care for their aging parents. By practicing self-care, caregivers can thrive in their caregiving role and find joy, meaning, and fulfillment in their relationships with their loved ones.

Chapter 6: Financial and Legal Considerations

6.1 Understanding Financial Planning for Aging Parents

Understanding financial planning for aging parents involves a comprehensive approach that encompasses various financial and legal considerations. As individuals age, they may encounter a range of challenges related to healthcare, housing, estate planning, and managing their finances. Caring for aging parents requires careful planning to ensure their well-being and financial security. Here are some of the key things to plan for:

1. Healthcare Costs and Insurance Coverage: Aging often brings about increased healthcare needs, including medical treatments, prescription drugs, and long-term care services. Understanding healthcare costs and insurance coverage is crucial for financial planning. Medicare, the federal health insurance program for people aged 65 and older, covers many healthcare services, but it does not cover all expenses. Supplemental insurance, such as Medigap policies or Medicare Advantage plans, can help fill the gaps in coverage. Additionally, long-term care insurance may be necessary to cover expenses related to nursing home care or assisted living facilities.

2. Estate Planning and Wills: Estate planning involves making arrangements for the distribution of assets and properties after death. It is essential for aging parents to have a will in place to ensure their wishes are carried out and to avoid disputes among family members. A will outlines how assets should be distributed

and may include provisions for guardianship of minor children, if applicable. In addition to a will, other estate planning documents such as trusts, powers of attorney, and advance directives should be considered. These documents allow aging parents to designate individuals to make financial and healthcare decisions on their behalf in the event of incapacity.

3. Financial Management and Budgeting: As aging parents transition into retirement, they may face changes in their income sources and expenses. It is essential to develop a comprehensive financial plan that accounts for retirement savings, Social Security benefits, pensions, and other sources of income. Budgeting becomes increasingly important to ensure that expenses are managed within the available resources. This may involve prioritizing essential expenses, such as housing and healthcare, while also setting aside funds for leisure activities and unexpected emergencies.

4. Long-Term Care Planning: Long-term care encompasses a range of services designed to help individuals with chronic illnesses or disabilities who need assistance with daily activities. Planning for long-term care is essential as it can be costly and may not be covered by traditional health insurance or government programs. Aging parents should explore options such as long-term care insurance, Medicaid planning, and self-funding through savings and investments. Long-term care preferences, including whether to receive care at home or in a facility, should be discussed and documented in advance.

5. Tax Planning and Retirement Accounts: Tax planning is an integral part of financial planning for aging parents. Understanding the tax

implications of retirement accounts, investment income, and estate transfers can help minimize tax liabilities and maximize savings. For example, distributions from retirement accounts such as 401(k)s and IRAs are typically subject to income tax, but there may be strategies to reduce taxes, such as Roth conversions or charitable contributions. Additionally, estate tax planning may be necessary for estates that exceed certain thresholds set by federal or state laws.

6. Legal Considerations and Documentation: Aging parents should review and update their legal documents regularly to ensure they reflect their current wishes and circumstances. This includes wills, trusts, powers of attorney, and advance directives for healthcare. It is also essential to keep important documents, such as birth certificates, marriage certificates, property deeds, and financial account information, organized and accessible. Legal considerations extend beyond estate planning to include issues such as guardianship, elder abuse, and incapacity planning. Consulting with an attorney who specializes in elder law can provide valuable guidance and assistance in navigating these complex legal matters.

Understanding financial planning for aging parents requires careful consideration of various financial and legal aspects. By proactively addressing healthcare costs, estate planning, financial management, long-term care, tax planning, and legal documentation, families can help ensure the well-being and financial security of their aging loved ones. Effective financial planning not only provides peace of mind for aging parents but also enables their caregivers to make informed decisions and navigate the complexities of aging with confidence.

6.2 Navigating Legal Issues and Documentation

Navigating legal issues and documentation is a critical component of financial planning when caring for aging parents. As individuals age, they may face various legal challenges related to estate planning, healthcare decision-making, guardianship, and asset management. Understanding and addressing these legal issues is essential to ensure the well-being and financial security of aging parents. These legal issues are as follows:

1. Estate Planning and Wills: Estate planning is the process of making arrangements for the distribution of assets and properties after death. For aging parents, having a comprehensive estate plan in place is essential to ensure their wishes are carried out and to avoid potential conflicts among family members. A will is a foundational document in estate planning that outlines how assets should be distributed upon death. Aging parents should work with an attorney to draft a will that accurately reflects their intentions and addresses any specific concerns or considerations, such as providing for minor children or charitable bequests. Additionally, other estate planning tools, such as trusts, can be used to manage assets and minimize taxes.

2. Powers of Attorney: Powers of attorney are legal documents that grant authority to another person to make financial or healthcare decisions on behalf of an individual. There are two main types of powers of attorney: financial and healthcare. A financial power of attorney allows an agent to manage financial matters, such as paying bills, managing investments, and selling property, on behalf of an aging parent who may become incapacitated. A healthcare

power of attorney, also known as a healthcare proxy or medical power of attorney, authorizes an agent to make medical decisions if the parent is unable to do so themselves. It is crucial for aging parents to carefully select agents they trust and to clearly communicate their wishes regarding financial and healthcare matters.

3. Advance Directives: Advance directives are legal documents that allow individuals to communicate their preferences for medical treatment in the event they become unable to make decisions for themselves. Common types of advance directives include living wills and healthcare proxies. A living will outlines the types of medical treatments a person does or does not want to receive in specific circumstances, such as life-sustaining treatments or palliative care. A healthcare proxy appoints a trusted individual to make medical decisions on behalf of the person if they are unable to do so. Advance directives ensure that aging parents' healthcare preferences are known and respected, reducing the burden on family members and healthcare providers during times of crisis.

4. Guardianship and Conservatorship: In some cases, aging parents may become incapacitated and unable to make decisions for themselves without having previously appointed an agent through a power of attorney. In such situations, family members may need to pursue guardianship or conservatorship proceedings to obtain legal authority to make decisions on behalf of the incapacitated parent. Guardianship typically involves decision-making authority over personal matters, such as healthcare and living arrangements, while conservatorship involves authority over financial matters. These legal proceedings can be complex and emotionally

challenging, so it is advisable to consult with an attorney who specializes in elder law to navigate the process effectively.

5. Long-Term Care Planning: Long-term care planning involves preparing for the possibility of needing assistance with activities of daily living due to aging, illness, or disability. Legal considerations play a crucial role in long-term care planning, particularly regarding eligibility for government benefits such as Medicaid. Medicaid is a joint federal and state program that provides healthcare coverage for individuals with limited income and assets, including coverage for long-term care services. However, Medicaid has strict eligibility requirements, including limits on income and assets. Long-term care planning may involve strategies to protect assets, such as transferring assets to trusts or purchasing long-term care insurance, to qualify for Medicaid while preserving financial security.

6. Legal Documentation and Record-Keeping: Proper documentation and record-keeping are essential aspects of legal planning for aging parents. Important documents to keep organized and accessible include birth certificates, marriage certificates, Social Security cards, passports, property deeds, financial account information, insurance policies, and estate planning documents. It is also crucial to maintain records of medical treatments, healthcare providers, and medications. Organizing and updating legal documents regularly can help ensure that aging parents' wishes are honored and that their affairs are managed effectively in accordance with applicable laws and regulations.

Navigating legal issues and documentation is integral to financial planning when caring for aging parents. By addressing estate planning, powers of attorney, advance directives, guardianship and conservatorship, long-term care planning, and legal documentation and record-keeping, families can help ensure the well-being and financial security of their aging loved ones. Consulting with experienced attorneys who specialize in elder law can provide valuable guidance and assistance in navigating the complex legal landscape associated with aging and incapacity. Effective legal planning not only protects aging parents' interests but also provides peace of mind for family members and caregivers as they navigate the challenges of aging together.

6.3 Accessing Government Benefits and Resources

Accessing government benefits and resources is a crucial aspect of financial planning when caring for aging parents. As individuals age, they may encounter increasing healthcare costs, long-term care needs, and other expenses that can strain their financial resources. Government programs and benefits can provide valuable support to help alleviate these financial burdens and ensure that aging parents have access to necessary services and resources. The following are some of the Government programs and benefits:

1. Social Security Benefits: Social Security is a federal program that provides retirement, disability, and survivor benefits to eligible individuals and their families. For aging parents who have worked and paid into the Social Security system, these benefits can be a

significant source of income during retirement. Eligibility for Social Security retirement benefits is based on factors such as age, work history, and earnings. The amount of benefits received depends on factors such as the individual's earnings history and the age at which they begin receiving benefits. It is essential for aging parents to understand their Social Security options and to make informed decisions about when to start receiving benefits, as delaying benefits can result in higher monthly payments.

2. Medicare: Medicare is a federal health insurance program for people aged 65 and older, as well as some younger individuals with disabilities or certain medical conditions. Medicare provides coverage for hospital care (Part A), medical services (Part B), and prescription drugs (Part D), as well as optional supplemental coverage (Part C) through Medicare Advantage plans. While Medicare covers many healthcare services, it does not cover all expenses, and beneficiaries may still be responsible for premiums, deductibles, coinsurance, and copayments. Understanding Medicare coverage options and potential out-of-pocket costs is essential for aging parents and their caregivers to effectively plan for healthcare expenses in retirement.

3. Medicaid: Medicaid is a joint federal and state program that provides healthcare coverage for individuals with limited income and resources. Unlike Medicare, which is primarily for older adults, Medicaid covers people of all ages, including children, pregnant women, and individuals with disabilities. Medicaid covers a wide range of medical services, including long-term care services such as nursing home care and home health care. Eligibility for Medicaid is based on income and asset limits, which vary by state. Medicaid

planning involves strategies to qualify for Medicaid while preserving assets, such as transferring assets to trusts or purchasing long-term care insurance. Aging parents and their caregivers should explore Medicaid eligibility requirements and available services to determine if Medicaid can help cover their healthcare needs.

4. Supplemental Security Income (SSI): Supplemental Security Income (SSI) is a federal program that provides cash assistance to low-income individuals aged 65 and older, as well as individuals with disabilities. SSI benefits are designed to help meet basic needs such as food, shelter, and clothing. Eligibility for SSI is based on income and resource limits, and benefit amounts vary depending on factors such as income, living arrangements, and marital status. SSI recipients may also be eligible for additional state and local assistance programs, such as Medicaid and food assistance programs. Aging parents who have limited income and resources may qualify for SSI benefits to supplement their financial resources and improve their quality of life.

5. Veterans Benefits: Veterans benefits are available to eligible veterans and their dependents through the U.S. Department of Veterans Affairs (VA). These benefits include healthcare services, disability compensation, pension benefits, education and training assistance, home loan guarantees, and burial benefits. Veterans who served on active duty and meet certain service requirements may qualify for VA healthcare services, which include medical treatment, preventive care, and long-term care services. Additionally, veterans with service-connected disabilities may be eligible for disability compensation, while low-income veterans aged 65 and older may qualify for VA pension benefits. Caregivers

of veterans may also be eligible for support services and benefits through programs such as the VA Caregiver Support Program.

6. Senior Nutrition and Assistance Programs: The federal government funds several nutrition and assistance programs aimed at supporting older adults' nutritional needs and promoting their independence and well-being. These programs include the Supplemental Nutrition Assistance Program (SNAP), formerly known as food stamps, which provides eligible individuals with electronic benefits to purchase food, as well as the Older Americans Act (OAA) nutrition programs, which include congregate meal sites, home-delivered meals, and nutrition counseling services. Additionally, the OAA funds a range of supportive services, such as transportation, caregiver support, and elder abuse prevention programs, to help older adults maintain their independence and quality of life.

7. Legal Assistance and Advocacy Services: Legal assistance and advocacy services are available to help aging parents and their caregivers navigate legal issues and access benefits and resources. Organizations such as the National Academy of Elder Law Attorneys (NAELA) and legal aid agencies provide legal advice, representation, and advocacy on a variety of legal matters, including estate planning, guardianship and conservatorship, Medicaid planning, and consumer protection. These services can help aging parents and their caregivers understand their rights and options under the law and ensure that they receive the benefits and services to which they are entitled.

Accessing government benefits and resources is an essential aspect of financial planning when caring for aging parents. By understanding the various programs available, including Social Security, Medicare, Medicaid, SSI, veterans benefits, senior nutrition and assistance programs, and legal assistance services, families can help ensure that aging parents receive the support they need to maintain their health, independence, and financial security. Effective utilization of government benefits and resources requires careful planning, coordination, and advocacy to navigate the complex eligibility requirements and application processes. By working with knowledgeable professionals and organizations, families can maximize their access to benefits and resources and provide the best possible care for their aging loved ones.

6.4 Planning for Long-Term Care Needs

Planning for long-term care needs is a critical aspect of financial and legal planning when caring for aging parents. Long-term care encompasses a range of services designed to assist individuals with chronic illnesses, disabilities, or cognitive impairments who need help with activities of daily living. As individuals age, the likelihood of needing long-term care increases, and the costs associated with long-term care can be substantial. Planning ahead for long-term care needs involves understanding the various care options available, evaluating financing options, and addressing legal considerations to ensure that aging parents receive the care they need while protecting their financial security. Below are some of the long-term care planning guide:

1. Understanding Long-Term Care Options: Long-term care can be provided in a variety of settings, including nursing homes, assisted living facilities, adult day care centers, and in-home care settings. Each option offers different levels of care and support, ranging from skilled nursing care in a nursing home to assistance with activities of daily living in an assisted living facility or home care setting. Aging parents and their caregivers should evaluate the pros and cons of each care option based on factors such as the individual's health needs, preferences, and financial resources. It is essential to consider factors such as the quality of care, availability of services, and cost when selecting a long-term care setting.

2. Assessing Long-Term Care Costs: Long-term care costs can vary widely depending on the type of care needed and the location of services. Nursing home care is typically the most expensive option, with costs averaging thousands of dollars per month. Assisted living and home care services may be less costly but can still strain the finances of aging parents and their families. It is essential to assess long-term care costs and develop a financial plan to cover these expenses. Long-term care insurance is one option to help offset the costs of care, providing coverage for services such as nursing home care, assisted living, and home care. Other financing options include personal savings, investments, retirement accounts, and government programs such as Medicaid.

3. Long-Term Care Insurance: Long-term care insurance is a type of insurance policy that provides coverage for long-term care services, such as nursing home care, assisted living, and home care. Long-term care insurance policies vary in terms of coverage, benefits, premiums, and eligibility requirements. When considering long-

term care insurance, aging parents and their caregivers should carefully review policy options and consider factors such as the cost of premiums, coverage limits, benefit triggers, and inflation protection. It is essential to purchase long-term care insurance while aging parents are still healthy and insurable, as premiums increase with age and health status.

4. Medicare and Medicaid Coverage: While Medicare provides coverage for some long-term care services, such as skilled nursing care following a hospital stay, it does not cover most long-term care expenses. Medicaid, on the other hand, is a joint federal and state program that provides coverage for long-term care services for eligible individuals with limited income and resources. Medicaid covers a wide range of long-term care services, including nursing home care, home health care, and personal care services. Eligibility for Medicaid is based on income and asset limits, which vary by state. Medicaid planning involves strategies to qualify for Medicaid while preserving assets, such as transferring assets to trusts or purchasing long-term care insurance.

5. Legal Considerations for Long-Term Care Planning: Long-term care planning involves various legal considerations that can affect aging parents' ability to access and pay for care. These legal considerations may include estate planning, advance directives, powers of attorney, guardianship and conservatorship, and Medicaid planning. It is essential for aging parents to have a comprehensive estate plan in place that addresses their long-term care preferences and ensures that their wishes are carried out in the event of incapacity or death. Advance directives, such as living wills and healthcare proxies, allow individuals to communicate their

preferences for medical treatment and designate a trusted individual to make healthcare decisions on their behalf if they become unable to do so themselves. Powers of attorney grant authority to another person to make financial and legal decisions on behalf of an aging parent who may become incapacitated. Guardianship and conservatorship proceedings may be necessary to obtain legal authority to make decisions on behalf of an incapacitated parent who has not appointed an agent through a power of attorney. Medicaid planning involves strategies to qualify for Medicaid while preserving assets, such as transferring assets to trusts or purchasing long-term care insurance.

6. Caregiver Support and Resources: Caring for aging parents with long-term care needs can be emotionally, physically, and financially challenging for caregivers. It is essential for caregivers to seek support and resources to help them navigate the caregiving journey and prevent burnout. Caregiver support services and resources are available through organizations such as the Family Caregiver Alliance, the National Alliance for Caregiving, and the Alzheimer's Association. These organizations offer information, education, support groups, respite care, and other services to help caregivers cope with the demands of caregiving and maintain their own health and well-being.

Planning for long-term care needs is an essential aspect of financial and legal planning when caring for aging parents. By understanding long-term care options, assessing long-term care costs, considering long-term care insurance, exploring Medicare and Medicaid coverage, addressing legal considerations, and seeking caregiver support and resources, families can help ensure that aging parents receive the care they need while protecting their financial security. Effective long-term care planning requires careful consideration of the individual's health needs, preferences, and financial resources, as well as coordination with healthcare providers, financial advisors, and legal professionals. By proactively planning for long-term care needs, families can provide peace of mind for aging parents and caregivers and navigate the challenges of aging with confidence.

Chapter 7: Cultivating Dignity and Respect

7.1 Upholding Dignity in Caregiving Practices

Upholding dignity in caregiving practices is a fundamental aspect of providing compassionate and respectful care to aging parents. Dignity encompasses the inherent worth and value of every individual, regardless of age, health status, or cognitive ability. When caring for aging parents, it is essential to recognize and honor their dignity by promoting autonomy, respecting their preferences and choices, and preserving their sense of identity and self-worth as follows:

1. Understand Dignity in Caregiving: Dignity in caregiving refers to treating aging parents with respect, compassion, and sensitivity, and recognizing their inherent worth and value as individuals. Upholding dignity involves honoring aging parents' autonomy, independence, and personal preferences, and preserving their sense of identity, self-worth, and self-respect. Dignity is not contingent on physical or cognitive abilities, but rather is an inherent aspect of every individual's humanity, deserving of recognition and respect in all aspects of caregiving.

2. Promoting Autonomy and Independence: Promoting autonomy and independence is essential for upholding dignity in caregiving practices. Aging parents should be encouraged and supported to make their own decisions, participate in activities of daily living, and maintain control over aspects of their lives to the greatest extent possible. Caregivers can promote autonomy by offering choices,

respecting preferences, and involving aging parents in decision-making about their care and daily routines.

3. Respecting Preferences and Choices: Respecting preferences and choices is another key aspect of upholding dignity in caregiving. Aging parents should be afforded the opportunity to express their preferences and make choices about their care, living environment, social activities, and end-of-life wishes. Caregivers should listen attentively to aging parents' preferences, respect their decisions, and involve them in discussions about their care and well-being.

4. Preserving Identity and Self-Worth: Preserving identity and self-worth is vital for maintaining dignity in caregiving practices. Aging parents should be treated as individuals with unique histories, personalities, and life experiences, rather than simply as recipients of care. Caregivers can preserve identity by acknowledging aging parents' accomplishments, interests, and values, and fostering opportunities for meaningful engagement and self-expression.

5. Strategies for Cultivating Dignity and Respect: Cultivating dignity and respect when caring for aging parents requires intentionality, compassion, and empathy. Some strategies for upholding dignity in caregiving practices include:

> a. Active Listening: Listen attentively to aging parents' concerns, preferences, and needs, and validate their experiences and feelings without judgment or criticism.

> b. Empowerment: Empower aging parents to make decisions about their care, daily routines, and lifestyle preferences,

and support them in maintaining control over aspects of their lives to the greatest extent possible.

c. Choice and Autonomy: Offer aging parents choices and opportunities to exercise autonomy in their daily lives, such as selecting clothing, meals, activities, and social interactions.

d. Respectful Communication: Communicate with aging parents respectfully, using clear, empathetic, and non-patronizing language, and honoring their dignity and worth in all interactions.

e. Privacy and Confidentiality: Respect aging parents' privacy and confidentiality by maintaining confidentiality of personal information, respecting personal space, and providing opportunities for private conversations and reflection.

f. Physical Care and Comfort: Provide physical care and comfort to aging parents with dignity and respect, ensuring that care practices are gentle, non-invasive, and responsive to individual preferences and needs.

g. Promotion of Social Interaction: Facilitate opportunities for aging parents to engage in social activities, connect with others, and maintain meaningful relationships and social connections.

h. Cultural Sensitivity: Recognize and respect the cultural backgrounds, beliefs, and traditions of aging parents, and incorporate cultural preferences and practices into caregiving routines and decision-making processes.

i. Advocacy and Empathy: Advocate for aging parents' rights, preferences, and needs, and demonstrate empathy and compassion in addressing their concerns, fears, and anxieties.

6. Impact of Dignity on Quality of Care and Well-Being: Upholding dignity in caregiving practices has a profound impact on the quality of care and well-being of both caregivers and aging parents. When caregivers prioritize dignity and respect in their interactions with aging parents, it fosters trust, mutual respect, and positive relationships built on empathy and understanding. This, in turn, contributes to improved communication, cooperation, and collaboration in caregiving, leading to better outcomes for aging parents and caregivers alike. Additionally, upholding dignity promotes a sense of purpose, meaning, and fulfillment in caregiving, as caregivers recognize the value and worth of their role in supporting aging parents with compassion and dignity.

7. Challenges and Barriers to Upholding Dignity in Caregiving: Despite the importance of upholding dignity in caregiving practices, there are challenges and barriers that may impede caregivers' ability to do so effectively. Some common challenges include:

a. Time Constraints: Caregivers may face time constraints and competing demands that limit their ability to provide personalized, dignified care to aging parents.

b. Burnout and Stress: Caregivers may experience burnout, stress, and emotional exhaustion from the demands of caregiving, making it difficult to maintain empathy and compassion in their interactions with aging parents.

c. Lack of Resources: Caregivers may lack access to resources, support services, and training opportunities that could enhance their ability to uphold dignity in caregiving practices.

d. Communication Barriers: Caregivers and aging parents may face communication barriers due to cognitive decline, language differences, or other factors, making it challenging to convey preferences, needs, and concerns effectively.

e. Systemic Issues: Systemic issues within the healthcare system, such as institutional practices, policies, and attitudes, may perpetuate disrespect, neglect, and violations of dignity in caregiving settings.

8. Overcoming Challenges and Promoting Dignity in Caregiving: Overcoming challenges and promoting dignity in caregiving requires a multi-faceted approach that addresses systemic issues, supports caregivers, and empowers aging parents.

Some strategies for overcoming challenges and promoting dignity in caregiving include:

a. Education and Training: Provide education and training opportunities for caregivers to enhance their knowledge, skills, and confidence in providing dignified care to aging parents.

b. Support Services: Offer support services, such as respite care, counseling, and caregiver support groups, to help caregivers cope with stress, burnout, and emotional challenges.

c. Advocacy and Policy Change: Advocate for policy changes and systemic reforms that promote dignity, respect, and person-centered care in caregiving settings, including long-term care facilities, hospitals, and community-based services.

d. Collaboration and Partnership: Foster collaboration and partnership between caregivers, healthcare providers, social services, and community organizations to coordinate care, share resources, and support aging parents and their families.

e. Cultural Competence: Provide cultural competence training and resources to caregivers and healthcare providers to enhance their understanding and appreciation of diverse cultural backgrounds, beliefs, and values, and promote culturally sensitive care practices.

f. Empowerment and Self-Care: Empower caregivers to prioritize their own well-being and self-care, and provide resources and support to help them manage stress, cope with burnout, and maintain resilience in their caregiving role.

Upholding dignity in caregiving practices is essential for promoting autonomy, respect, and quality of life for aging parents. By recognizing and honoring aging parents' inherent worth and value as individuals, caregivers can cultivate a culture of dignity and respect in caregiving settings, fostering positive relationships, communication, and collaboration.

Despite the challenges and barriers that may arise, caregivers can overcome these obstacles and promote dignity in caregiving through education, support, advocacy, and empowerment. Ultimately, upholding dignity in caregiving practices contributes to the well-being and dignity of both caregivers and aging parents, enriching the caregiving experience and enhancing the quality of care provided.

7.2 Respecting Autonomy and Independence

Respecting autonomy and independence is a cornerstone of cultivating dignity and respect when caring for aging parents. Autonomy refers to the right of individuals to make their own decisions and choices about their lives, while independence refers to the ability to carry out activities of daily living and make choices without undue influence or interference from others. When caregivers respect the autonomy and independence of aging parents, they honor their inherent worth and dignity as individuals, promote their sense of self-worth and self-esteem, and empower them to live with dignity. Some helpful tips are as follows:

1. Understand Autonomy and Independence: Autonomy and independence are essential aspects of human dignity and well-being, enabling individuals to make choices and decisions that reflect their values, preferences, and priorities. As aging parents grow older, they may face physical, cognitive, or functional changes that impact their ability to maintain independence and autonomy in their daily lives. However, it is essential to recognize that autonomy and independence are not solely dependent on physical or cognitive abilities, but rather encompass the right of individuals to make choices and decisions about their lives based on their own values, beliefs, and preferences.

2. Promoting Autonomy in Decision-Making: Promoting autonomy in decision-making involves respecting aging parents' right to make choices and decisions about their care, living arrangements, medical treatment, and end-of-life wishes. Caregivers can promote autonomy by:

> a. Encouraging Participation: Encouraging aging parents to actively participate in discussions about their care, treatment options, and goals of care, and involving them in decision-making processes to the extent possible given their cognitive and functional abilities.

b. Providing Information: Providing aging parents with accurate, unbiased information about their health conditions, treatment options, and prognosis, and supporting them in making informed decisions that align with their values and preferences.

c. Respecting Choices: Respecting aging parents' choices and decisions, even if they differ from the caregiver's preferences or expectations, and honoring their right to autonomy and self-determination in all aspects of their lives.

d. Offering Support: Offering emotional support, reassurance, and validation to aging parents as they navigate difficult decisions and choices about their care and well-being, and empowering them to advocate for their own needs and preferences.

3. Supporting Independence in Activities of Daily Living: Supporting independence in activities of daily living involves helping aging parents maintain their ability to carry out daily tasks, routines, and responsibilities to the greatest extent possible. Caregivers can support independence by:

a. Encouraging Self-Care: Encouraging aging parents to engage in self-care activities, such as grooming, dressing, bathing, and meal preparation, and providing assistance and support as needed to promote independence and autonomy.

b. Adapting the Environment: Adapting the home environment to promote safety, accessibility, and independence for aging parents, such as installing grab bars, handrails, and ramps, and removing obstacles or hazards that may impede mobility or function.

c. Assistive Devices and Technology: Providing aging parents with assistive devices and technology to enhance their independence and autonomy, such as walkers, canes, hearing aids, and smartphone apps for medication reminders or emergency assistance.

d. Encouraging Social Engagement: Encouraging aging parents to engage in social activities, hobbies, and interests that promote independence, social connection, and a sense of purpose and fulfillment.

4. Respecting Autonomy and Independence in End-of-Life Care: Respecting autonomy and independence is particularly important in the context of end-of-life care, as aging parents face difficult decisions about their treatment preferences, goals of care, and end-of-life wishes. Caregivers can respect autonomy and independence in end-of-life care by:

a. Facilitating Advance Care Planning: Facilitating discussions about advance care planning with aging parents, including preferences for medical treatment, resuscitation, artificial nutrition and hydration, and end-of-life care, and documenting these preferences in advance directives, such as living wills and healthcare proxies.

b. Honoring End-of-Life Wishes: Honoring aging parents' end-of-life wishes and preferences, even if they differ from the caregiver's own beliefs or values, and ensuring that care decisions are guided by the aging parent's autonomy and self-determination.

c. Providing Comfort and Palliative Care: Providing comfort-focused care and palliative interventions that prioritize symptom management, pain relief, and emotional support, and respect aging parents' wishes for comfort and dignity in the final stages of life.

d. Respecting Cultural and Spiritual Beliefs: Respecting aging parents' cultural and spiritual beliefs and practices regarding death and dying, and incorporating these beliefs into end-of-life care planning and decision-making processes.

5. Benefits of Respecting Autonomy and Independence: Respecting autonomy and independence in caregiving has numerous benefits for both aging parents and caregivers. Some of these benefits include:

a. Enhanced Dignity and Self-Worth: Respecting autonomy and independence promotes a sense of dignity, self-worth, and self-esteem in aging parents, as they are empowered to make choices and decisions that reflect their values, preferences, and priorities.

b. Improved Quality of Life: Supporting independence in activities of daily living enhances the quality of life for aging parents, enabling them to maintain a sense of purpose, and control over their lives, despite physical or cognitive limitations.

c. Positive Caregiver Relationships: Respecting autonomy and independence fosters positive relationships between caregivers and aging parents, built on mutual respect, trust, and collaboration, and enhances communication, cooperation, and partnership in caregiving.

d. Reduced Caregiver Stress: Supporting autonomy and independence in caregiving reduces caregiver stress, burnout, and burden, as aging parents are able to contribute to their own care and well-being, and caregivers feel supported in their efforts to promote independence and dignity.

6. Challenges and Barriers to Respecting Autonomy and Independence: Despite the importance of respecting autonomy and independence in caregiving, there are challenges and barriers that may impede caregivers' ability to do so effectively. Some common challenges include:

a. Role Reversal and Power Imbalance: Caregivers may struggle with feelings of power imbalance and role reversal when assuming responsibility for the care of aging parents, leading to conflicts over decision-making and autonomy.

b. Cognitive Decline and Decision-Making Capacity: Aging parents may experience cognitive decline or impairment that affects their decision-making capacity, making it difficult for caregivers to respect their autonomy and independence in decision-making processes.

c. Cultural and Familial Expectations: Cultural and familial expectations regarding caregiving roles and responsibilities may conflict with principles of autonomy and independence, leading to tension and conflict within the family.

d. Healthcare System Constraints: Constraints within the healthcare system, such as limited resources, time constraints, and institutional policies, may limit caregivers' ability to respect autonomy and independence in caregiving practices.

7. Overcoming Challenges and Promoting Autonomy and Independence: Overcoming challenges and promoting autonomy and independence in caregiving requires a multi-faceted approach that addresses systemic issues, supports caregivers, and empowers aging parents. Some strategies for overcoming challenges and promoting autonomy and independence include:

a. Education and Training: Provide education and training opportunities for caregivers to enhance their understanding of autonomy and independence in caregiving, and develop skills for promoting these principles in practice.

b. Support Services: Offer support services, such as respite care, counseling, and caregiver support groups, to help caregivers cope with stress, burnout, and emotional challenges, and provide resources and guidance for promoting autonomy and independence in caregiving.

c. Communication and Collaboration: Foster open communication and collaboration between caregivers, aging parents, and healthcare providers to facilitate shared decision-making, honor aging parents' preferences and choices, and promote autonomy and independence in caregiving practices.

d. Advocacy and Policy Change: Advocate for policy changes and systemic reforms that support autonomy and independence in caregiving, including policies that promote person-centered care, advance care planning, and shared decision-making.

e. Empowerment and Self-Care: Empower caregivers to prioritize their own well-being and self-care, and provide resources and support to help them manage stress, cope with burnout, and maintain resilience in their caregiving role.

Respecting autonomy and independence is essential for promoting dignity, self-worth, and well-being in aging parents, and fostering positive relationships and communication between caregivers and aging parents. By recognizing aging parents' right to make choices and decisions about their care and well-being, and supporting their independence in activities of daily living, caregivers can cultivate a culture of respect, autonomy, and dignity in caregiving relationships. Despite the challenges and barriers that may arise, caregivers can overcome these obstacles and promote autonomy and independence through education, support, advocacy, and empowerment, ultimately enhancing the quality of life and care for aging parents and caregivers alike.

7.3 Advocating for the Rights of Aging Parents

Advocating for the rights of aging parents is a critical component of cultivating dignity and respect when caring for them. Aging parents, like all individuals, have inherent rights that deserve to be upheld and protected as they age. These rights include autonomy, dignity, independence, and the right to receive quality care and support that respects their preferences and promotes their well-being. However, aging parents may face various challenges and vulnerabilities that can threaten their rights, such as ageism, discrimination, neglect, and abuse. Caregivers play a crucial role in advocating for the rights of aging parents, ensuring that they are treated with dignity, respect, and compassion in all aspects of their care and daily lives. Some helpful tips are as follows:

1. Understand the Rights of Aging Parents: Aging parents, like all individuals, have inherent rights that deserve to be respected and protected as they age. Some key rights of aging parents include:

> a. Autonomy: The right to make decisions about their care, living arrangements, medical treatment, and end-of-life wishes based on their own values, preferences, and priorities.

b. Dignity: The right to be treated with respect, compassion, and sensitivity, and to have their inherent worth and value as individuals recognized and honored.

c. Independence: The right to maintain control over aspects of their lives, carry out activities of daily living, and make choices without undue influence or interference from others.

d. Safety and Security: The right to receive care and support that ensures their safety, security, and well-being, and protects them from harm, neglect, and abuse.

e. Quality of Care: The right to receive high-quality, person-centered care that meets their individual needs, preferences, and goals, and promotes their physical, emotional, and spiritual well-being.

2. Challenges Facing Aging Parents: Aging parents may face various challenges and vulnerabilities that can threaten their rights and well-being as they age. Some common challenges facing aging parents include:

a. Ageism: Ageism refers to stereotypes, prejudices, and discrimination against individuals based on their age, and can lead to marginalization, devaluation, and mistreatment of aging parents in healthcare, social, and community settings.

b. Healthcare Disparities: Aging parents may experience disparities in access to healthcare services, including preventive care, screenings, and treatment, which can impact their health outcomes and quality of life.

c. Financial Exploitation: Aging parents may be at risk of financial exploitation, fraud, or abuse, particularly if they are vulnerable due to cognitive decline, isolation, or dependence on others for care and support.

d. Elder Abuse and Neglect: Aging parents may experience elder abuse or neglect in various forms, including physical, emotional, financial, or sexual abuse, as well as neglect of basic needs, such as food, shelter, and medical care.

e. End-of-Life Issues: Aging parents may face complex decisions and challenges related to end-of-life care, including advance care planning, palliative care, hospice care, and decision-making about life-sustaining treatments and interventions.

3. The Role of Caregivers in Advocacy: Caregivers play a crucial role in advocating for the rights of aging parents, ensuring that their voices are heard, their needs are met, and their rights are respected and protected. Some key roles and responsibilities of caregivers in advocacy include:

a. Empowerment: Empowering aging parents to assert their rights, voice their preferences, and advocate for themselves in healthcare, social, and community settings.

b. Education: Educating aging parents about their rights, resources, and options for care and support, and providing information and guidance to help them navigate the complexities of the healthcare system and aging process.

c. Communication: Communicating effectively with healthcare providers, social workers, and other professionals on behalf of aging parents, advocating for their needs, preferences, and concerns, and ensuring that they receive respectful, compassionate care.

d. Collaboration: Collaborating with aging parents, family members, and other caregivers to develop care plans, make decisions about their care and well-being, and address any issues or challenges that arise.

e. Monitoring and Oversight: Monitoring the quality of care and services received by aging parents, and advocating for improvements or changes as needed to ensure that their rights and well-being are protected.

f. Reporting Abuse or Neglect: Reporting suspected cases of elder abuse or neglect to appropriate authorities, such as adult protective services or law enforcement agencies, and advocating for interventions to address safety concerns and protect aging parents from harm.

4. Strategies for Effective Advocacy: Effective advocacy for the rights of aging parents requires a proactive, collaborative, and multi-faceted approach. Some strategies for effective advocacy include:

a. Know Your Rights: Educate yourself and aging parents about their rights, legal protections, and resources available to them, including local, state, and federal laws governing elder rights and protections.

b. Build Relationships: Build positive, collaborative relationships with healthcare providers, social workers, and other professionals involved in the care of aging parents, and advocate for their needs, preferences, and concerns in a respectful and assertive manner.

c. Document Concerns: Keep detailed records of interactions, observations, and concerns related to the care and well-being of aging parents, including any instances of mistreatment, neglect, or abuse, and use this documentation to advocate for improvements or changes as needed.

d. Seek Support: Seek support from family members, friends, support groups, and advocacy organizations that specialize in elder rights and protections, and collaborate with them to advocate for systemic changes and reforms to address issues facing aging parents.

e. Stay Informed: Stay informed about current issues, trends, and developments in elder rights and protections, and advocate for policy changes and reforms that promote the rights, dignity, and well-being of aging parents at the local, state, and national levels.

f. Be Persistent: Be persistent and tenacious in advocating for the rights of aging parents, even in the face of obstacles, challenges, or resistance, and continue to speak out and take action to ensure that their voices are heard and their rights are respected and protected.

5. Impact of Advocacy on Quality of Care and Well-Being: Advocating for the rights of aging parents has a profound impact on the quality of care and well-being of aging parents, caregivers, and families. Some of the benefits of advocacy include:

a. Improved Quality of Care: Advocacy helps ensure that aging parents receive high-quality, person-centered care that meets their individual needs, preferences, and goals, and promotes their physical, emotional, and spiritual well-being.

b. Enhanced Dignity and Respect: Advocacy promotes a culture of dignity, respect, and compassion in caregiving settings, ensuring that aging parents are treated with respect, kindness, and sensitivity in all aspects of their care and daily lives.

c. Empowerment and Self-Determination: Advocacy empowers aging parents to assert their rights, voice their preferences, and make decisions about their care and well-being based on their own values, beliefs, and priorities.

d. Prevention of Abuse and Neglect: Advocacy helps prevent elder abuse and neglect by raising awareness, identifying risk factors, and implementing interventions to address safety concerns and protect aging parents from harm.

e. Support for Caregivers: Advocacy provides support and resources for caregivers, enabling them to navigate the complexities of caregiving, address challenges and concerns, and advocate effectively on behalf of aging parents.

6. Challenges and Barriers to Advocacy: Despite the importance of advocacy for the rights of aging parents, there are challenges and barriers that may impede caregivers' ability to advocate effectively. Some common challenges include:

a. Power Imbalance: Caregivers may face power imbalances and conflicts of interest in advocating for the rights of aging parents, particularly if they are also responsible for their care and decision-making.

b. Communication Barriers: Communication barriers, such as language differences, cultural differences, or cognitive impairments, may hinder effective advocacy for aging parents, making it difficult to convey their needs, preferences, and concerns to healthcare providers and other professionals.

c. Systemic Issues: Systemic issues within the healthcare system, such as limited resources, time constraints, and institutional policies, may create barriers to effective advocacy for aging parents, making it challenging to address issues or concerns in a timely and meaningful manner.

d. Resistance to Change: Resistance to change, inertia, or apathy among healthcare providers, social workers, and other professionals may hinder efforts to advocate for the rights of aging parents, requiring caregivers to be persistent and tenacious in their advocacy efforts.

7. Overcoming Challenges and Promoting Advocacy: Overcoming challenges and promoting advocacy for the rights of aging parents requires a concerted effort from caregivers, families, healthcare providers, policymakers, and community stakeholders. Some strategies for overcoming challenges and promoting advocacy include:

a. Education and Training: Provide education and training opportunities for caregivers, healthcare providers, and other professionals to enhance their understanding of elder rights and protections, and develop skills for effective advocacy.

b. Collaboration and Partnership: Foster collaboration and partnership between caregivers, families, healthcare providers, policymakers, advocacy organizations, and community stakeholders to address issues and concerns facing aging parents, and advocate for systemic changes and reforms to promote their rights and well-being.

c. Legislation and Policy Change: Advocate for legislation and policy changes at the local, state, and national levels that promote the rights, dignity, and well-being of aging parents, including laws governing elder abuse prevention, long-term care services, and healthcare decision-making.

d. Community Outreach and Awareness: Raise awareness about elder rights and protections through community outreach, education campaigns, and media advocacy, and empower aging parents and caregivers to advocate for themselves and others in similar situations.

e. Support Services and Resources: Provide support services and resources for aging parents and caregivers, such as legal assistance, counseling, and advocacy support, to help them navigate the complexities of aging and caregiving, and advocate effectively for their rights and well-being.

Advocating for the rights of aging parents is essential for promoting dignity, respect, and well-being in caregiving relationships, and ensuring that aging parents receive the care and support they need and deserve as they age. By empowering aging parents to assert their rights, voice their preferences, and make decisions about their care and well-being, and advocating effectively on their behalf, caregivers can help protect their rights, preserve their dignity, and enhance their quality of life in the later stages of life. Despite the challenges and barriers that may arise, caregivers can overcome these obstacles and promote advocacy through education, collaboration, legislation, community outreach, and support services, ultimately making a positive difference in the lives of aging parents and their families.

7.4 Celebrating the Legacy of Aging Loved Ones

Celebrating the legacy of an aging loved one is a profound way to honor their life, accomplishments, and contributions, while also cultivating dignity and respect in the caregiving journey. As aging parents navigate the later stages of life, it becomes increasingly important to recognize and commemorate their legacy, preserving their memories, stories, and values for future generations. Celebrating the legacy of aging loved ones not only affirms their inherent worth and dignity but also fosters a sense of connection, meaning, and gratitude within the family and community. The following tips may be helpful:

1. Understand the Legacy of Aging Loved Ones: The legacy of aging loved ones encompasses the collective impact of their life experiences, values, beliefs, and contributions on the lives of others. It reflects the enduring influence and significance of their actions, relationships, and accomplishments, and provides a framework for understanding their identity, purpose, and meaning in the world. The legacy of aging loved ones may include:

a. Personal Accomplishments: Achievements, milestones, and successes in various domains of life, such as career, education, family, and community involvement.

b. Values and Beliefs: Core values, principles, and beliefs that guide their actions and decisions, and shape their relationships, priorities, and perspectives.

c. Life Lessons and Wisdom: Insights, lessons, and wisdom gained from life experiences, challenges, and triumphs, and shared with others as a source of guidance and inspiration.

d. Impact on Others: Influence, support, and encouragement provided to family members, friends, colleagues, and community members, and the lasting impression left on their lives and hearts.

2. Significance of Celebrating Legacy: Celebrating the legacy of aging loved ones is a meaningful way to honor their life journey, affirm their inherent worth and dignity, and express gratitude for their presence and contributions. Some key reasons for celebrating legacy include:

a. Honoring Identity: Celebrating legacy acknowledges the unique identity and worth of aging loved ones, recognizing their individuality, accomplishments, and impact on the world.

b. Preserving Memories and Stories: Celebrating legacy preserves memories, stories, and experiences of aging loved ones, ensuring that their life journey is remembered, valued, and passed down to future generations.

c. Fostering Connection and Bonding: Celebrating legacy brings family members and loved ones together to share stories, memories, and reflections, fostering connection, understanding, and appreciation within the family unit.

d. Promoting Healing and Closure: Celebrating legacy provides an opportunity for healing and closure as aging loved ones reflect on their life journey, reconcile past experiences, and find peace and fulfillment in their legacy.

e. Inspiring Future Generations: Celebrating legacy inspires future generations to learn from the experiences, values, and lessons of aging loved ones, and to carry forward their legacy of love, resilience, and compassion in their own lives and relationships.

3. Strategies for Celebrating Legacy: There are many ways to celebrate the legacy of aging loved ones, each tailored to their unique interests, preferences, and values. Some strategies for celebrating legacy include:

a. Storytelling and Reminiscing: Gather family members and loved ones to share stories, memories, and anecdotes about aging loved ones, highlighting their achievements, experiences, and impact on others.

b. Creating Memory Books or Scrapbooks: Compile photographs, mementos, and memorabilia into memory books or scrapbooks that capture the life journey and legacy of aging loved ones, and provide a tangible keepsake for future generations.

c. Recording Oral Histories: Record oral histories and interviews with aging loved ones, capturing their voices, perspectives, and insights on life experiences, family history, and personal values.

d. Organizing Legacy Events: Plan special events or gatherings to celebrate the legacy of aging loved ones, such as milestone birthdays, anniversaries, or family reunions, and incorporate meaningful rituals, traditions, or activities that honor their life and contributions.

e. Creating Legacy Projects: Collaborate on legacy projects or initiatives that reflect the passions, interests, or values of aging loved ones, such as community service projects, charitable donations, or creative endeavors that leave a lasting impact on others.

f. Documenting Family History: Document the family history and genealogy of aging loved ones, tracing their ancestry, heritage, and cultural traditions, and preserving this legacy for future generations to cherish and learn from.

g. Honoring Life Milestones: Honor life milestones and achievements of aging loved ones, such as graduations, career accomplishments, or retirement, with special ceremonies, tributes, or awards that recognize their contributions and significance.

4. Impact of Celebrating Legacy on Caregiving Relationships: Celebrating the legacy of aging loved ones has a transformative impact on caregiving relationships, enhancing communication, understanding, and connection between caregivers and aging parents. Some of the benefits of celebrating legacy on caregiving relationships include:

a. Enhanced Communication and Bonding: Celebrating legacy fosters open communication, empathy, and understanding between caregivers and aging loved ones, as they share stories, memories, and reflections on their life journey.

b. Validation and Recognition: Celebrating legacy validates the worth and significance of aging loved ones, affirming their identity, accomplishments, and impact on others, and promoting a sense of self-worth and dignity in caregiving relationships.

c. Healing and Closure: Celebrating legacy provides an opportunity for healing and closure for both caregivers and aging loved ones, as they reflect on their shared experiences, reconcile past conflicts or regrets, and find peace and acceptance in their legacy.

d. Strengthened Family Connections: Celebrating legacy brings family members and loved ones together to honor and celebrate aging loved ones, strengthening family bonds, traditions, and connections across generations.

e. Inspiration and Legacy Building: Celebrating legacy inspires caregivers and family members to carry forward the values, lessons, and legacy of aging loved ones in their own lives and relationships, creating a ripple effect of love, resilience, and compassion in the world.

5. Overcoming Challenges in Celebrating Legacy: While celebrating the legacy of aging loved ones is a meaningful and rewarding experience, it may also present challenges and obstacles that caregivers must navigate. Some common challenges in celebrating legacy include:

a. Health Limitations: Aging loved ones may face health limitations or mobility issues that impact their ability to participate in legacy celebration activities, requiring caregivers to adapt plans and accommodations to meet their needs.

b. Communication Barriers: Communication barriers, such as cognitive decline or language differences, may hinder effective communication and storytelling between caregivers and aging loved ones, necessitating patience, empathy, and creativity in facilitating meaningful connections.

c. Family Dynamics: Family dynamics, conflicts, or tensions may arise during legacy celebration activities, leading to disagreements or misunderstandings that require patience, understanding, and conflict resolution strategies to address.

d. Emotional Challenges: Legacy celebration may evoke a range of emotions for caregivers and aging loved ones, including joy, gratitude, sadness, or nostalgia, requiring sensitivity, support, and validation in processing and expressing these emotions.

6. Promoting Dignity and Respect through Legacy Celebration: Celebrating the legacy of aging loved ones is a powerful way to promote dignity and respect in caregiving relationships, affirming their worth, identity, and contributions in the later stages of life. Some ways in which legacy celebration promotes dignity and respect include:

a. Honoring Individuality: Celebrating legacy honors the individuality and uniqueness of aging loved ones, recognizing their inherent worth and dignity as individuals with a rich and meaningful life journey.

b. Valuing Life Experiences: Celebrating legacy values the life experiences, wisdom, and insights of aging loved ones, acknowledging their contributions and impact on others, and affirming their significance and relevance in the world.

c. Fostering Connection and Understanding: Celebrating legacy fosters connection, empathy, and understanding between caregivers and aging loved ones, as they share stories, memories, and reflections on their shared experiences and relationships.

d. Promoting Self-Worth and Validation: Celebrating legacy promotes a sense of self-worth and validation in aging loved ones, affirming their identity, accomplishments, and contributions, and recognizing the value of their presence and impact on others.

e. Leaving a Lasting Legacy: Celebrating legacy leaves a lasting legacy of love, resilience, and compassion in caregiving relationships, inspiring future generations to honor and carry forward the values, lessons, and legacy of aging loved ones in their own lives and relationships.

Celebrating the legacy of aging loved ones is a powerful way to honor their life, accomplishments, and contributions, while also cultivating dignity and respect in caregiving relationships. By recognizing and commemorating the legacy of aging loved ones, caregivers affirm their inherent worth and dignity, preserve their memories and stories for future generations, and foster connection, understanding, and gratitude within the family and community. Despite the challenges and obstacles that may arise, caregivers can overcome these barriers and promote legacy celebration through empathy, creativity, and collaboration, ultimately creating a lasting legacy of love, resilience, and compassion in caregiving relationships and beyond.

Chapter 8: Finding Support and Resources

8.1 Identifying Community Support Services

Identifying community support services is crucial when caring for aging parents as it facilitates finding the necessary support and resources to meet their needs effectively. Community support services encompass a wide range of programs, organizations, and resources designed to assist caregivers and aging parents in navigating the challenges of aging and caregiving. These services offer practical assistance, emotional support, information, and resources to help caregivers and aging parents maintain their well-being, independence, and quality of life. A few tips regarding community support services are as follows:

Understanding Community Support Services

Community support services encompass a diverse array of programs, organizations, and resources available within local communities to assist caregivers and aging parents. These services are designed to address various aspects of aging and caregiving, including healthcare, social support, financial assistance, housing, transportation, and legal services. Some common types of community support services include:

1. Adult Day Programs: Daytime programs that offer supervised activities, socialization, and support services for aging adults, providing respite for caregivers and stimulating engagement for aging parents.

2. Home Care Services: In-home care services that provide assistance with activities of daily living, such as personal care, meal preparation, medication management, and light housekeeping, to help aging parents remain independent and safe in their own homes.

3. Respite Care: Temporary care services that allow caregivers to take a break from their caregiving responsibilities and recharge, while aging parents receive care and supervision from trained professionals in a residential or community-based setting.

4. Support Groups: Peer-led or professionally facilitated groups that offer emotional support, education, and information to caregivers and aging parents, allowing them to share experiences, strategies, and resources with others facing similar challenges.

5. Transportation Services: Transportation assistance programs that provide door-to-door or escorted transportation for aging parents to medical appointments, grocery shopping, social outings, and other essential destinations.

6. Legal and Financial Assistance: Legal and financial counseling services that offer guidance and support to caregivers and aging parents on issues such as estate planning, advance care planning, guardianship, insurance, benefits eligibility, and fraud prevention.

7. Senior Centers: Community centers or facilities that offer a wide range of programs, activities, and services for aging adults, including fitness classes, educational workshops, social events, and recreational opportunities.

8. Meal Delivery Programs: Meal delivery services that provide nutritious, home-delivered meals to aging parents who are unable to cook or shop for themselves, ensuring they have access to proper nutrition and food security.

9. Caregiver Education and Training: Educational workshops, seminars, and training programs that offer caregivers practical skills, strategies, and resources for managing the challenges of caregiving, improving communication, and enhancing self-care.

Importance of Identifying Community Support Services

Identifying community support services is essential for caregivers and aging parents as it provides access to the resources, assistance, and support needed to navigate the complexities of aging and caregiving effectively. Some reasons why identifying community support services is important include:

1. Meeting Diverse Needs: Community support services offer a range of programs and resources tailored to the diverse needs and preferences of caregivers and aging parents, ensuring they receive personalized support and assistance that meets their unique circumstances.

2. Enhancing Quality of Life: Community support services enhance the quality of life for caregivers and aging parents by providing practical assistance, emotional support, and social connections that promote well-being, independence, and engagement.

3. Reducing Caregiver Burden: Community support services alleviate caregiver burden by offering respite care, support groups, and other services that provide relief from caregiving responsibilities and prevent burnout, exhaustion, and isolation.

4. Promoting Aging in Place: Community support services enable aging parents to age in place safely and independently by providing home care services, transportation assistance, and other resources that support aging in the familiar environment of their own homes and communities.

5. Improving Access to Care: Community support services improve access to healthcare, social services, and other resources for aging parents by providing transportation, advocacy, and assistance with navigating the healthcare system and accessing benefits and entitlements.

6. Empowering Caregivers: Community support services empower caregivers by offering education, training, and resources that enhance their caregiving skills, knowledge, and confidence, and help them advocate for the needs and preferences of aging parents.

Strategies for Accessing Community Support Services

Accessing community support services requires proactive research, outreach, and collaboration with local organizations, agencies, and providers. Some strategies for accessing community support services include:

1. Research and Information Gathering: Conduct research online, through local directories, or by contacting community agencies and organizations to identify available support services, eligibility criteria, and contact information.

2. Networking and Referrals: Reach out to healthcare providers, social workers, and other professionals for referrals to community support services and resources that may benefit caregivers and aging parents.

3. Attend Community Events and Workshops: Attend community events, workshops, and seminars hosted by local organizations and agencies to learn about available support services, connect with service providers, and access resources and information.

4. Contact Local Agencies and Organizations: Contact local agencies and organizations, such as area agencies on aging, senior centers, and nonprofit organizations, to inquire about available support services, eligibility requirements, and enrollment procedures.

5. Utilize Online Resources and Helplines: Explore online resources, websites, and helplines that provide information and assistance on aging and caregiving-related topics, including support groups, educational materials, and referral services.

6. Meet with Care Coordinators or Case Managers: Schedule meetings with care coordinators or case managers who can assess the needs of caregivers and aging parents, develop care plans, and coordinate access to community support services and resources.

Benefits of Leveraging Community Support Services

Leveraging community support services offers numerous benefits for caregivers and aging parents, enhancing their well-being, resilience, and quality of life. Some of the benefits of leveraging community support services include:

1. Enhanced Caregiver Well-Being: Community support services provide practical assistance, emotional support, and respite care that alleviate caregiver stress, burnout, and burden, and promote self-care, resilience, and well-being.

2. Improved Health Outcomes: Community support services improve health outcomes for aging parents by facilitating access to healthcare, medication management, nutrition services, and preventive care, and reducing the risk of hospitalizations and complications.

3. Social Engagement and Connection: Community support services offer opportunities for socialization, engagement, and connection for aging parents, reducing social isolation, loneliness, and depression, and promoting a sense of belonging and purpose.

4. Financial Assistance and Benefits: Community support services provide financial assistance, benefits counseling, and advocacy services that help caregivers and aging parents access entitlements, benefits, and resources to support their care needs and expenses.

5. Enhanced Quality of Life: Community support services enhance the quality of life for caregivers and aging parents by addressing

their physical, emotional, social, and spiritual needs, and promoting independence, dignity, and self-determination.

6. Peace of Mind and Security: Community support services provide peace of mind and security for caregivers and aging parents, knowing that they have access to the resources, assistance, and support needed to navigate the challenges of aging and caregiving effectively.

Overcoming Challenges in Accessing Community Support Services

Despite the benefits of community support services, caregivers and aging parents may encounter challenges and barriers in accessing these services. Some common challenges include:

1. Limited Availability: Community support services may be limited in availability or capacity, particularly in rural or underserved areas, making it difficult to access needed resources and assistance.

2. Financial Barriers: Some community support services may have eligibility criteria or cost-sharing requirements that pose financial barriers for caregivers and aging parents, limiting their ability to access needed support.

3. Navigating the System: Navigating the complex healthcare and social service system can be challenging for caregivers and aging parents, particularly if they are unfamiliar with available resources, eligibility requirements, and enrollment procedures.

4. Stigma and Shame: Stigma, shame, and cultural beliefs may prevent caregivers and aging parents from seeking or accepting help from community support services, leading to reluctance to access available resources and support.

5. Language and Cultural Barriers: Language and cultural barriers may hinder access to community support services for caregivers and aging parents who are non-English speakers or from diverse cultural backgrounds, requiring culturally competent and language-accessible services and resources.

6. Transportation and Accessibility: Transportation and accessibility issues may limit access to community support services for aging parents with mobility impairments or transportation limitations, requiring accommodations and assistance to overcome these barriers.

Promoting Awareness and Engagement in Community Support Services

Promoting awareness and engagement in community support services requires collaboration, outreach, and education to ensure that caregivers and aging parents are aware of available resources and how to access them effectively. Some strategies for promoting awareness and engagement in community support services include:

1. Education and Outreach: Provide educational materials, workshops, and outreach events to raise awareness about available community support services, eligibility criteria, and enrollment procedures.

2. Community Partnerships: Forge partnerships with local organizations, agencies, and businesses to promote community support services and collaborate on outreach efforts to reach underserved populations.

3. Cultural Competency and Language Access: Ensure that community support services are culturally competent and accessible to diverse populations, including non-English speakers and individuals from diverse cultural backgrounds.

4. Technology and Telehealth: Utilize technology and telehealth platforms to expand access to community support services for caregivers and aging parents, particularly in remote or underserved areas where in-person services may be limited.

5. Peer Support and Mentoring: Offer peer support groups, mentoring programs, and outreach ambassadors to connect caregivers and aging parents with others who have similar experiences and can provide guidance, support, and encouragement.

6. Advocacy and Policy Change: Advocate for policy changes and systemic reforms that promote access to community support services, address barriers and disparities in service delivery, and enhance funding and resources for aging and caregiving-related programs and initiatives.

Identifying community support services is essential for caregivers and aging parents as it provides access to the resources, assistance, and support needed to navigate the challenges of aging and caregiving effectively. By leveraging community support services, caregivers and aging parents can enhance their well-being, resilience, and quality of life, and promote independence, dignity, and self-determination in the later stages of life. Despite the challenges and barriers that may arise, caregivers and aging parents can overcome these obstacles and access community support services through proactive research, outreach, collaboration, and advocacy, ultimately creating a supportive and compassionate community that empowers and uplifts caregivers and aging parents alike.

8.2 Accessing Respite Care and Support Groups

Accessing respite care and support groups is crucial for caregivers when caring for aging parents as it provides essential relief, emotional support, and resources to manage the challenges of caregiving effectively. Respite care offers temporary relief for caregivers, allowing them to take breaks, recharge, and attend to their own needs while aging parents receive care and supervision from trained professionals. Support groups offer caregivers opportunities to connect with others facing similar challenges, share experiences, strategies, and resources, and receive emotional support, validation, and encouragement. Some of the points mentioned in this section are similar to those mentioned in the previous section on "Identifying community support services."

Respite care provides temporary relief for caregivers by offering short-term care and supervision for aging parents, allowing caregivers to take breaks, attend to their own needs, and prevent burnout and exhaustion. Respite care services may be provided in-home, through adult day programs, or in residential care facilities, and may include personal care, supervision, companionship, and recreational activities for aging parents. On the other hand, support groups are peer-led or professionally facilitated groups that offer emotional support, education, and resources to caregivers facing the challenges of caregiving. Support groups provide opportunities for caregivers to connect with others, share experiences, insights, and strategies, and receive validation, encouragement, and practical advice in a supportive and understanding environment.

Importance of Accessing Respite Care and Support Groups

1. Preventing Caregiver Burnout: Accessing respite care allows caregivers to take breaks and recharge, preventing burnout, exhaustion, and compassion fatigue, and promoting their physical, emotional, and mental well-being.

2. Improving Caregiver Health Outcomes: Respite care supports caregiver health outcomes by reducing stress, anxiety, and depression, and promoting self-care, resilience, and coping strategies, ultimately improving caregiver health and quality of life.

3. Enhancing Care Recipient Well-Being: Respite care enhances the well-being of care recipients by providing them with socialization, engagement, and stimulation, and ensuring they receive quality care and supervision while caregivers take breaks and attend to their own needs.

4. Promoting Connection and Support: Accessing support groups promotes connection, validation, and support for caregivers, allowing them to share experiences, insights, and resources, and receive emotional support, encouragement, and practical advice from others facing similar challenges.

5. Reducing Social Isolation: Support groups reduce social isolation and loneliness for caregivers by providing opportunities for connection, camaraderie, and belonging with others who understand their experiences and challenges, fostering a sense of community and support.

6. Enhancing Coping and Problem-Solving Skills: Support groups enhance caregivers' coping and problem-solving skills by providing them with access to diverse perspectives, insights, and strategies for managing the challenges of caregiving, and empowering them to navigate obstacles and setbacks more effectively.

Strategies for Finding and Utilizing Respite Care and Support Groups

1. Research and Information Gathering: Conduct research online, through local directories, or by contacting community agencies and organizations to identify available respite care services, support groups, and resources for caregivers.

2. Networking and Referrals: Reach out to healthcare providers, social workers, and other professionals for referrals to respite care services and support groups that may benefit caregivers and aging parents.

3. Attend Community Events and Workshops: Attend community events, workshops, and seminars hosted by local organizations and agencies to learn about available respite care services, support groups, and resources for caregivers.

4. Contact Local Agencies and Organizations: Contact local agencies and organizations, such as Area Agencies on Aging, senior centers, and nonprofit organizations, to inquire about available respite care services, support groups, and caregiver resources in the community.

5. Utilize Online Resources and Helplines: Explore online resources, websites, and helplines that provide information and assistance on respite care services, support groups, and caregiver resources, including directories, educational materials, and referral services.

6. Participate in Caregiver Education and Training: Participate in caregiver education and training programs, workshops, and seminars that offer information, resources, and support for caregivers, and provide opportunities to connect with others facing similar challenges.

7. Meet with Care Coordinators or Case Managers: Schedule meetings with care coordinators or case managers who can assess the needs of caregivers and aging parents, develop care plans, and coordinate access to respite care services, support groups, and other resources.

Benefits of Incorporating Respite Care and Support Group Participation

1. Enhanced Caregiver Well-Being: Incorporating respite care and support group participation enhances caregiver well-being by providing opportunities for rest, relaxation, and self-care, and offering emotional support, validation, and encouragement from peers and professionals.

2. Reduced Caregiver Stress: Respite care and support group participation reduce caregiver stress, anxiety, and depression by providing relief from caregiving responsibilities, fostering social connections, and enhancing coping and problem-solving skills.

3. Improved Care Recipient Outcomes: Incorporating respite care and support group participation improves care recipient outcomes by ensuring they receive quality care and supervision during caregivers' breaks, promoting their socialization, engagement, and well-being, and reducing the risk of neglect or abuse.

4. Promotion of Connection and Support: Respite care and support group participation promote connection and support for caregivers by fostering relationships, camaraderie, and understanding with others who share similar experiences and challenges, and providing a safe space to share insights, strategies, and resources.

5. Enhanced Coping and Adaptation: Respite care and support group participation enhance caregivers' coping and adaptation skills by providing access to diverse perspectives, insights, and strategies for

managing the challenges of caregiving, and empowering them to navigate obstacles and setbacks more effectively.

6. Increased Socialization and Engagement: Respite care and support group participation increase socialization and engagement for caregivers, reducing social isolation and loneliness, and fostering a sense of belonging and community with others who understand their experiences and struggles.

Overcoming Challenges in Accessing Respite Care and Support Groups

1. Limited Availability: Respite care services and support groups may be limited in availability or capacity, particularly in rural or underserved areas, making it difficult for caregivers to access needed resources and support.

2. Financial Barriers: Some respite care services may have eligibility criteria or cost-sharing requirements that pose financial barriers for caregivers, limiting their ability to access needed relief and support.

3. Navigating the System: Navigating the complex healthcare and social service system can be challenging for caregivers, particularly if they are unfamiliar with available resources, eligibility requirements, and enrollment procedures for respite care services and support groups.

4. Stigma and Shame: Stigma, shame, and cultural beliefs may prevent caregivers from seeking or accepting help from respite care

services and support groups, leading to reluctance to access available resources and support.

5. Transportation and Accessibility: Transportation and accessibility issues may limit access to respite care services and support groups for caregivers and aging parents with mobility impairments or transportation limitations, requiring accommodations and assistance to overcome these barriers.

Promoting Awareness and Engagement in Respite Care and Support Groups

1. Education and Outreach: Provide educational materials, workshops, and outreach events to raise awareness about the importance of respite care and support group participation for caregivers, and provide information on available resources and how to access them effectively.

2. Community Partnerships: Forge partnerships with local organizations, agencies, and businesses to promote respite care services and support groups, and collaborate on outreach efforts to reach underserved populations and raise awareness about available resources.

3. Cultural Competency and Language Access: Ensure that respite care services and support groups are culturally competent and accessible to diverse populations, including non-English speakers and individuals from diverse cultural backgrounds.

4. Technology and Telehealth: Utilize technology and telehealth platforms to expand access to respite care services and support groups for caregivers, particularly in remote or underserved areas where in-person services may be limited.

5. Peer Support and Mentoring: Offer peer support groups, mentoring programs, and outreach ambassadors to connect caregivers with others who have similar experiences and can provide guidance, support, and encouragement.

Accessing respite care and support groups is essential for caregivers when caring for aging parents as it provides essential relief, emotional support, and resources to manage the challenges of caregiving effectively. By incorporating respite care and support group participation into the caregiving journey, caregivers can enhance their well-being, resilience, and quality of life, and promote independence, dignity, and self-determination for themselves and their aging parents. Despite the challenges and barriers that may arise, caregivers can overcome these obstacles and access respite care and support groups through proactive research, outreach, and collaboration.

8.3 Utilizing Technology and Innovative Solutions

Utilizing technology and innovative solutions is increasingly important for caregivers when caring for aging parents as it provides access to a wide range of support, resources, and tools to enhance caregiving efficiency, effectiveness, and quality of life. Technology and innovation offer caregivers opportunities to streamline communication, coordination, and monitoring of care, access information and resources remotely, and engage in virtual support networks and communities.

Importance of Utilizing Technology and Innovative Solutions

1. Enhancing Caregiver Efficiency: Utilizing technology and innovative solutions enhances caregiver efficiency by automating tasks, streamlining communication, and providing access to information and resources remotely, allowing caregivers to manage caregiving responsibilities more effectively.

2. Improving Care Coordination: Technology and innovative solutions improve care coordination by facilitating communication and collaboration among caregivers, healthcare providers, and other stakeholders, ensuring seamless coordination of care and support for aging parents.

3. Promoting Remote Monitoring: Technology enables remote monitoring of aging parents' health, safety, and well-being through devices such as wearables, sensors, and remote monitoring systems, allowing caregivers to track vital signs, activity levels, and medication adherence from a distance.

4. Accessing Information and Resources: Technology provides caregivers with access to a wealth of information, resources, and support services online, including educational materials, training programs, support groups, and telehealth services, empowering caregivers with knowledge and resources to meet their needs.

5. Engaging in Virtual Support Networks: Technology enables caregivers to engage in virtual support networks and communities, connecting with others who share similar experiences, challenges, and concerns, and providing mutual support, validation, and encouragement in a supportive and understanding environment.

Examples of Technologies and Solutions for Caregivers

1. Telehealth and Telemedicine: Telehealth and telemedicine platforms allow caregivers to access virtual healthcare services, consultations, and appointments remotely, reducing the need for in-person visits and providing convenient access to healthcare professionals and specialists.

2. Mobile Apps: Mobile apps offer a wide range of caregiving tools and resources, including medication reminders, care coordination platforms, symptom trackers, and emergency response systems, allowing caregivers to manage caregiving tasks and responsibilities more efficiently.

3. Wearable Devices: Wearable devices such as smartwatches, fitness trackers, and medical alert systems provide caregivers with real-time monitoring of aging parents' health metrics, activity levels, and safety alerts, enabling early detection of health issues and emergencies.

4. Smart Home Technology: Smart home technology, including voice-activated assistants, smart thermostats, and home security systems, enhances safety, comfort, and accessibility for aging

parents, and provides caregivers with remote monitoring and control of home environments.

5. Telecommunication Tools: Telecommunication tools such as video conferencing platforms, messaging apps, and social media networks facilitate communication and connection between caregivers, aging parents, and other family members, regardless of geographic distance or time constraints.

6. Robotic Assistants: Robotic assistants and devices offer assistance with daily tasks and activities of daily living for aging parents, including medication management, mobility assistance, and household chores, reducing caregiver burden and promoting independence.

7. Virtual Reality and Cognitive Training: Virtual reality and cognitive training programs offer cognitive stimulation and rehabilitation for aging parents with cognitive impairments or dementia, improving cognitive function, memory, and quality of life.

8. Caregiver Support Platforms: Caregiver support platforms and online communities provide caregivers with access to peer support, educational resources, expert advice, and caregiving tools and services, facilitating collaboration, learning, and empowerment.

Strategies for Incorporating Technology into Caregiving Practices

1. Assess Needs and Preferences: Assess caregivers' needs, preferences, and comfort levels with technology to identify appropriate tools and solutions that align with their caregiving goals.

2. Research and Explore Options: Research and explore available technologies and solutions for caregiving, including online reviews, demonstrations, and consultations with healthcare professionals or technology experts, to identify suitable options for caregivers and aging parents.

3. Provide Training and Support: Provide caregivers with training and support on how to use technology and innovative solutions effectively, including tutorials, user guides, and technical assistance, to ensure successful implementation and adoption of new tools and practices.

4. Integrate Technology into Care Plans: Integrate technology into care plans and routines for aging parents, incorporating tools and solutions that enhance communication, monitoring, and support for caregivers and aging parents, and align with their care needs and preferences.

5. Promote Collaboration and Communication: Promote collaboration and communication among caregivers, aging parents, and healthcare providers through technology-enabled platforms and tools, facilitating information sharing, care coordination, and decision-making.

6. Monitor and Evaluate Use: Monitor and evaluate caregivers' use of technology and innovative solutions over time, soliciting feedback, assessing outcomes, and making adjustments as needed to optimize effectiveness and address any barriers or challenges.

7. Stay Informed and Up-to-Date: Stay informed and up-to-date on advancements in technology and innovative solutions for caregiving, including attending workshops, webinars, and conferences, and participating in online forums and communities, to remain abreast of emerging trends and opportunities.

Benefits and Challenges of Leveraging Technology in Caregiving

Benefits of leveraging technology in caregiving include:
1. Enhanced caregiver efficiency and effectiveness.
2. Improved care coordination and communication.
3. Remote monitoring of aging parents' health and safety.
4. Access to information, resources, and support services.
5. Engagement in virtual support networks and communities.

Challenges of leveraging technology in caregiving include:
1. Technological barriers and accessibility issues for aging parents.
2. Privacy and security concerns related to data sharing and confidentiality.
3. Cost of technology and ongoing maintenance and support.
4. Learning curve and resistance to adopting new tools and practices.
5. Digital divide and disparities in access to technology and internet connectivity.

Promoting Awareness and Engagement in Technology and Innovative Solutions

1. Education and Outreach: Provide education and outreach to caregivers, aging parents, and healthcare professionals on the

benefits and opportunities of utilizing technology and innovative solutions in caregiving, and offer training and support to facilitate adoption and integration into caregiving practices.

2. Community Partnerships: Forge partnerships with technology companies, healthcare organizations, and community agencies to promote awareness and access to technology-enabled solutions for caregivers, and collaborate on initiatives to address barriers and enhance adoption and utilization.

3. Advocacy and Policy Change: Advocate for policy changes and systemic reforms that promote access to technology and innovative solutions for caregivers, address barriers and disparities in technology adoption, and enhance funding and resources for caregiving-related technology initiatives and programs.

Utilizing technology and innovative solutions is increasingly important for caregivers when caring for aging parents as it provides access to a wide range of support, resources, and tools to enhance caregiving efficiency, effectiveness, and quality of life. By incorporating technology into caregiving practices, caregivers can improve care coordination, access information and resources remotely, engage in virtual support networks and communities, and promote independence and well-being for aging parents. Despite the challenges and barriers that may arise, caregivers can overcome these obstacles and leverage technology in the caregiving journey through proactive research, exploration, training, and collaboration, ultimately enhancing the caregiving experience and outcomes for caregivers and aging parents alike.

8.4 Self-help Strategies for Caregiver Well-being

Self-help strategies for caregiver well-being are essential for maintaining the health, resilience, and quality of life of caregivers when caring for aging parents. These strategies encompass a range of practices, activities, and interventions that caregivers can implement to manage stress, promote self-care, and enhance their physical, emotional, and mental well-being. By prioritizing their own needs and engaging in self-help strategies, caregivers can better cope with the challenges of caregiving, prevent burnout and exhaustion, and sustain their ability to provide effective care and support for aging parents.

Importance of Self-Help Strategies for Caregiver Well-being

1. Preventing Burnout and Exhaustion: Self-help strategies prevent burnout and exhaustion by providing caregivers with tools and resources to manage stress, set boundaries, and prioritize self-care, ensuring they can sustain their caregiving role over the long term.

2. Enhancing Resilience and Coping Skills: Self-help strategies enhance caregivers' resilience and coping skills by promoting adaptive coping mechanisms, problem-solving skills, and emotional regulation techniques, enabling them to navigate the challenges of caregiving more effectively.

3. Promoting Physical and Emotional Health: Self-help strategies promote caregivers' physical and emotional health by encouraging healthy lifestyle habits, stress management techniques, and self-

care practices that reduce the risk of chronic illness, mental health issues, and caregiver-related health problems.

4. Improving Caregiving Effectiveness: Caregiver well-being directly impacts caregiving effectiveness, as caregivers who prioritize their own well-being are better able to provide compassionate, attentive care and support for aging parents, resulting in improved outcomes and quality of life for both caregivers and care recipients.

5. Fostering Positive Relationships: Self-help strategies foster positive relationships and communication between caregivers and aging parents by reducing stress, tension, and conflict, and promoting empathy, patience, and understanding in caregiving relationships.

6. Enhancing Overall Quality of Life: Self-help strategies enhance caregivers' overall quality of life by promoting balance, fulfillment, and satisfaction in their lives, beyond their caregiving responsibilities, and fostering a sense of purpose, meaning, and resilience in the face of challenges.

Examples of Self-Help Strategies and Activities

1. Self-care Practices: Engage in self-care practices such as regular exercise, healthy eating, adequate sleep, and relaxation techniques (e.g., deep breathing, meditation, yoga) to promote physical and emotional well-being.

2. Social Support Networks: Seek support from friends, family members, support groups, and online communities to share

experiences, receive validation and encouragement, and foster connections with others who understand the challenges of caregiving.

3. Time Management and Boundaries: Set boundaries and prioritize tasks to manage time effectively, balance caregiving responsibilities with personal needs and interests, and prevent overwhelm and burnout.

4. Stress Management Techniques: Practice stress management techniques such as mindfulness, progressive muscle relaxation, guided imagery, and journaling to reduce stress, anxiety, and tension, and promote relaxation and emotional regulation.

5. Hobbies and Interests: Engage in hobbies, interests, and activities that bring joy, fulfillment, and relaxation, and provide opportunities for self-expression, creativity, and personal growth outside of caregiving responsibilities.

6. Seeking Professional Help: Seek professional help from therapists, counselors, or mental health professionals to address caregiver-related stress, anxiety, depression, or other mental health concerns, and develop coping strategies and resilience skills.

7. Education and Training: Participate in caregiver education and training programs, workshops, and seminars to learn about caregiving best practices, communication skills, stress management techniques, and self-care strategies.

8. Respite Care and Support Services: Utilize respite care services, support groups, and community resources to take breaks, and access emotional support, validation, and encouragement from peers and professionals.

Strategies for Incorporating Self-Help into Caregiving Practices:

1. Assess Needs and Priorities: Assess caregivers' needs, priorities, and preferences for self-help strategies and activities to identify suitable options that align with their well-being goals and caregiving circumstances.

2. Create a Self-Care Plan: Develop a personalized self-care plan that outlines specific self-help strategies and activities to promote caregiver well-being, including goals, action steps, and resources for implementation and evaluation.

3. Schedule Regular Self-Care Time: Schedule regular time for self-care activities and practices, incorporating them into daily routines or weekly schedules to ensure consistency and commitment to prioritizing caregiver well-being.

4. Set Realistic Goals and Expectations: Set realistic goals and expectations for self-help efforts, recognizing that caregiving responsibilities may fluctuate and require flexibility in self-care practices and priorities.

5. Communicate Needs and Boundaries: Communicate needs and boundaries with family members, friends, and other stakeholders involved in caregiving to enlist support, set expectations, and

negotiate arrangements for sharing caregiving responsibilities and self-care time.

6. Seek Support and Accountability: Seek support and accountability from trusted individuals, such as friends, family members, or support group members, to help maintain motivation, consistency, and commitment to self-help efforts.

7. Monitor Progress and Adjustments: Monitor progress and adjustments in self-help efforts over time, evaluating the effectiveness of strategies and activities, identifying areas for improvement or refinement, and making necessary adjustments to enhance well-being and resilience.

Benefits of Prioritizing Caregiver Well-being

1. Improved Physical Health: Prioritizing caregiver well-being improves physical health outcomes by reducing stress, enhancing immune function, and promoting healthy lifestyle habits such as regular exercise and adequate sleep.

2. Enhanced Emotional Resilience: Caregiver well-being enhances emotional resilience and coping skills, enabling caregivers to manage stress, navigate challenges, and maintain a positive outlook in their caregiving role.

3. Better Caregiving Effectiveness: Caregiver well-being directly impacts caregiving effectiveness by promoting attentiveness, compassion, and patience in caregiving interactions, resulting in improved outcomes and quality of life for aging parents.

4. Reduced Risk of Burnout and Compassion Fatigue: Prioritizing caregiver well-being reduces the risk of burnout and compassion fatigue by providing caregivers with tools and resources to manage stress, set boundaries, and engage in self-care practices that sustain their ability to provide effective care and support.

5. Enhanced Quality of Life for Caregivers and Aging Parents: Caregiver well-being enhances the overall quality of life for caregivers and aging parents by fostering balance, fulfillment, and satisfaction in caregivers' lives, and promoting positive caregiving relationships and experiences for all involved.

Challenges and Barriers to Self-Help for Caregiver Well-being

1. Time Constraints: Caregivers may face time constraints and competing demands that make it challenging to prioritize self-help strategies and activities amidst caregiving responsibilities and other obligations.

2. Guilt and Obligation: Caregivers may experience guilt or obligation related to prioritizing their own needs and well-being over those of their aging parents, leading to reluctance to engage in self-care practices or seek support and resources for themselves.

3. Financial Constraints: Financial constraints may limit caregivers' ability to access self-help resources and support services, such as respite care or counseling, particularly if they are not covered by insurance or are cost-prohibitive.

4. Social Isolation: Caregivers may experience social isolation and loneliness due to the demands of caregiving, making it difficult to engage in self-help activities or seek support from others, particularly if they lack a strong support network or community resources.

Promoting Awareness and Engagement in Self-Help Strategies for Caregiver Well-being

1. Education and Outreach: Provide education and outreach to caregivers, aging parents, and healthcare professionals on the importance of self-help strategies for caregiver well-being, and offer resources, tools, and support to facilitate implementation and integration into caregiving practices.

2. Community Support and Resources: Develop and promote community support networks and resources for caregivers, including support groups, workshops, and online forums, to foster connection, validation, and encouragement, and provide opportunities for peer support and learning.

3. Advocacy and Policy Change: Advocate for policy changes and systemic reforms that support caregiver well-being, including access to respite care services, caregiver support programs, and financial assistance for caregiving-related expenses, and enhance funding and resources for caregiver wellness initiatives and programs.

Self-help strategies for caregiver well-being are essential for maintaining the health, resilience, and quality of life of caregivers when caring for aging parents. By prioritizing their own needs and engaging in self-help practices, caregivers can better cope with the challenges of caregiving, prevent burnout and exhaustion, and sustain their capacity to provide effective care and support for aging parents. Despite the challenges and barriers that may arise, caregivers can overcome these obstacles and prioritize their well-being through proactive assessment, planning, and implementation of self-help strategies and activities, ultimately enhancing their ability to thrive in their caregiving role and promote positive outcomes for themselves and their aging parents.

Chapter 9: End-of-Life Care and Decision Making

9.1 Having Difficult Conversations about End-of-Life Wishes

Having difficult conversations about end-of-life wishes is a crucial aspect of end-of-life care and decision-making when caring for aging parents. As individuals age, it becomes increasingly important to discuss and document their preferences for medical treatment, life-sustaining interventions, and other end-of-life care decisions. These conversations can be emotionally challenging but are essential for ensuring that aging parents' wishes are honored and respected, and that caregivers are prepared to make informed decisions in the event of a medical crisis. Below are helpful tips:

1. Understand the Importance of End-of-Life Conversations: Having difficult conversations about end-of-life wishes is essential for several reasons. Firstly, it allows aging parents to communicate their preferences for medical treatment and end-of-life care, ensuring that their wishes are known and respected by caregivers and healthcare providers. Secondly, it provides an opportunity for families to discuss sensitive topics such as life support, resuscitation, and hospice care, reducing the likelihood of conflicts and misunderstandings during times of crisis. Thirdly, it empowers aging parents to make informed decisions about their healthcare and end-of-life care, giving them a sense of control and dignity as they approach the end of life.

2. Initiating End-of-Life Conversations: Initiating end-of-life conversations with aging parents can be challenging, but it is

essential to approach these discussions with sensitivity, empathy, and respect. Here are some strategies for initiating end-of-life conversations:

a. Choose an appropriate time and place: Select a quiet and comfortable setting where everyone feels relaxed and can speak openly without interruptions.

b. Start the conversation gently: Begin by expressing your love and concern for your aging parents and explaining why you think it is important to have this conversation.

c. Ask open-ended questions: Encourage your aging parents to share their thoughts, feelings, and wishes about end-of-life care without judgment or pressure.

d. Listen actively: Listen attentively to what your aging parents have to say, and validate their feelings and concerns. Avoid interrupting or imposing your own views.

e. Respect their autonomy: Acknowledge that your aging parents have the right to make their own healthcare decisions and express their wishes accordingly. Offer support and assistance, but ultimately respect their autonomy and choices.

3. Discussing End-of-Life Wishes and Preferences: When discussing end-of-life wishes with aging parents, it is essential to cover a range of topics related to medical treatment, comfort care, and advance care planning. Some key areas to address include:

a. Preferences for life-sustaining treatments: Discuss your aging parents' preferences for interventions such as cardiopulmonary resuscitation (CPR), mechanical ventilation, and artificial nutrition and hydration.

b. Quality of life considerations: Explore your aging parents' values, beliefs, and priorities regarding quality of life and what matters most to them in their final days and weeks.

c. Palliative and hospice care options: Talk about the benefits of palliative care and hospice care in providing comfort, pain relief, and emotional support at the end of life.

d. Spiritual and emotional needs: Address your aging parents' spiritual and emotional needs, and explore how they would like these needs to be met during their final days and hours.

e. Funeral and burial preferences: Discuss your aging parents' preferences for funeral arrangements, burial or cremation, and any other end-of-life rituals or traditions that are important to them.

4. Documenting End-of-Life Wishes and Advance Directives: Once end-of-life wishes have been discussed and clarified, it is essential to document these preferences in writing through advance directives, such as living wills and healthcare proxies. Advance directives allow aging parents to specify their preferences for medical treatment and appoint a trusted individual to make healthcare decisions on their behalf if they become unable to do so themselves. It is essential to review and update advance directives regularly to ensure that they accurately reflect aging parents' current wishes and preferences. Additionally, copies of advance directives should be distributed to healthcare providers, family members, and other relevant individuals to ensure that everyone is aware of the aging parents' wishes and can act accordingly in the event of a medical crisis.

5. Involving Healthcare Providers and Other Professionals: Healthcare providers, social workers, and other professionals can play a valuable role in facilitating end-of-life conversations and advance care planning for aging parents. These professionals can provide information, guidance, and support to help families navigate difficult decisions and ensure that aging parents' wishes are honored. Healthcare providers can also help clarify medical options, prognosis, and potential outcomes, enabling aging parents and their families to make informed decisions about end-of-life care. It is essential to involve healthcare providers and other professionals early in the process and to maintain open communication throughout the caregiving journey.

6. Navigating Family Dynamics and Conflicts: End-of-life conversations can sometimes lead to conflicts or disagreements among family members, especially if there are differences of opinion regarding medical treatment or end-of-life care. It is essential to approach these discussions with sensitivity and empathy, recognizing that everyone may have different perspectives and priorities. Here are some strategies for navigating family dynamics and conflicts:

   a. Foster open communication: Encourage family members to express their thoughts, feelings, and concerns openly and respectfully, and listen actively to what each person has to say.

   b. Seek common ground: Focus on areas of agreement and shared values, and look for solutions that honor aging parents' wishes while addressing family members' concerns.

   c. Involve a neutral third party: Consider involving a mediator, counselor, or other neutral third party to facilitate discussions and help resolve conflicts in a constructive and respectful manner.

   d. Respect autonomy and individual choices: Recognize that each family member has the right to express their own preferences and make their own healthcare decisions, and respect their autonomy and individual choices accordingly.

7. Seeking Support and Resources: End-of-life conversations can be emotionally challenging for aging parents and their caregivers, and it is essential to seek support and resources to help cope with the emotional and practical aspects of end-of-life care and decision-making. Support services and resources are available through organizations such as the National Hospice and Palliative Care Organization, the Conversation Project, and local hospice programs. These organizations offer information, education, support groups, and other services to help families navigate end-of-life care with compassion, dignity, and peace of mind.

Having difficult conversations about end-of-life wishes is an essential aspect of end-of-life care and decision-making when caring for aging parents. By initiating these conversations with sensitivity, empathy, and respect, families can ensure that aging parents' wishes are known and honored, and that caregivers are prepared to make informed decisions in the event of a medical crisis. Advance care planning allows aging parents to express their preferences for medical treatment and end-of-life care, empowering them to make choices that reflect their values, beliefs, and priorities. By documenting end-of-life wishes through advance directives and involving healthcare providers and other professionals, families can ensure that aging parents receive the care and support they need to live their final days with dignity, comfort, and peace.

9.2 Understanding Advance Directives and Healthcare Proxy

Understanding advance directives and healthcare proxies is crucial for end-of-life care and decision-making when caring for aging parents. Advance directives are legal documents that allow individuals to specify their preferences for medical treatment and appoint a healthcare proxy to make healthcare decisions on their behalf if they become unable to do so themselves. These documents help ensure that aging parents' wishes are known and respected, and that their healthcare preferences are honored during times of illness or incapacity. The following are helping tips:

1. Importance of Advance Directives and Healthcare Proxies: Advance directives and healthcare proxies play a crucial role in end-of-life care and decision-making for aging parents. These documents allow individuals to express their preferences for medical treatment and appoint a trusted individual to make healthcare decisions on their behalf if they become unable to do so themselves. By documenting their wishes in advance, aging parents can ensure that their healthcare preferences are known and respected by caregivers and healthcare providers, reducing the likelihood of conflicts or misunderstandings during times of illness or incapacity. Advance directives and healthcare proxies empower aging parents to make informed decisions about their healthcare and end-of-life care, giving them a sense of control and autonomy as they age.

2. Understanding Advance Directives: Advance directives are legal documents that allow individuals to specify their preferences for medical treatment and end-of-life care in advance. There are several types of advance directives, including:

> a. Living Will: A living will is a written document that outlines an individual's preferences for medical treatment and end-of-life care, such as preferences for life-sustaining treatments, resuscitation, and artificial nutrition and hydration. A living will typically takes effect when the individual is unable to communicate their wishes due to illness or incapacity.

> b. Healthcare Power of Attorney: As earlier mentioned, a healthcare power of attorney, also known as a healthcare proxy or medical power of attorney, is a legal document that appoints a trusted individual to make healthcare decisions on behalf of the individual if they become unable to do so themselves. The healthcare proxy is responsible for making medical treatment decisions that are consistent with the individual's wishes and best interests.

> c. Do-Not-Resuscitate (DNR) Order: A Do-Not-Resuscitate (DNR) order is a medical order that instructs healthcare providers not to attempt cardiopulmonary resuscitation (CPR) in the event of cardiac arrest. A DNR order is typically signed by a physician and is included in the individual's medical records.

3. Appointing a Healthcare Proxy: Appointing a healthcare proxy is an important step in advance care planning for aging parents. A healthcare proxy is a trusted individual who is authorized to make healthcare decisions on behalf of the individual if they become unable to do so themselves. When appointing a healthcare proxy, aging parents should choose someone who knows their values, beliefs, and preferences regarding medical treatment and end-of-life care, and who is willing and able to fulfill the responsibilities of the role. It is essential to have open and honest discussions with the chosen healthcare proxy about the individual's wishes and preferences, and to ensure that they understand their role and responsibilities as a healthcare decision-maker.

4. Completing a Living Will: Completing a living will is another important aspect of advance care planning for aging parents. A living will allows individuals to document their preferences for medical treatment and end-of-life care in writing, ensuring that their wishes are known and respected by caregivers and healthcare providers. When completing a living will, aging parents should carefully consider their preferences regarding life-sustaining treatments, resuscitation, artificial nutrition and hydration, and other medical interventions. It is essential to be specific and clear about these preferences, and to review and update the living will regularly to ensure that it accurately reflects the individual's current wishes and preferences.

5. Legal Requirements and Considerations: Advance directives and healthcare proxies are legal documents that must meet certain requirements to be valid and enforceable. These requirements may vary by state, but typically include:

> a. Legal Capacity: The individual must have legal capacity to execute the advance directive, meaning they must be of sound mind and able to understand the nature and consequences of their decisions.

> b. Witnesses: Advance directives must be witnessed by one or more individuals who are not related to the individual and who do not stand to benefit from the individual's estate. Some states may require a notary public to witness the document as well.

> c. Documentation: Advance directives should be properly documented and stored in a safe and accessible location, such as with the individual's healthcare provider, family members, and/or legal representative. Copies of the advance directives should also be provided to the individual's healthcare providers to ensure that their wishes are known and respected.

6. Role of Advance Directives in End-of-Life Care: Advance directives play a crucial role in end-of-life care by ensuring that aging parents' wishes for medical treatment and end-of-life care are known and respected by caregivers and healthcare providers. In the event of illness or incapacity, advance directives guide healthcare decisions and help prevent unnecessary interventions or treatments that may

not align with the individual's preferences. By documenting their wishes in advance, aging parents can provide clarity and guidance to their healthcare proxy and other decision-makers, enabling them to make informed decisions that reflect the individual's values, beliefs, and preferences.

7. Navigating Difficult Decisions and Conflicts: End-of-life care decisions can sometimes be difficult and emotionally challenging for aging parents and their families, especially if there are disagreements or conflicts regarding medical treatment and end-of-life care. In such situations, advance directives and healthcare proxies can help provide clarity and guidance, ensuring that the individual's wishes are honored and respected. It is essential to approach these decisions with sensitivity, empathy, and respect for the individual's autonomy and dignity, and to involve healthcare providers, social workers, and other professionals as needed to facilitate discussions and resolve conflicts in a constructive and respectful manner.

8. Educating and Empowering Aging Parents: Educating and empowering aging parents to make informed decisions about advance directives and healthcare proxies is an essential aspect of end-of-life care planning. Aging parents should be encouraged to learn about advance care planning and the importance of documenting their wishes for medical treatment and end-of-life care. They should also be encouraged to discuss these preferences with their healthcare providers, family members, and other relevant individuals, and to review and update their advance directives regularly to ensure that they accurately reflect their current wishes and preferences.

Understanding advance directives and healthcare proxies is essential for end-of-life care and decision-making when caring for aging parents. These legal documents allow individuals to specify their preferences for medical treatment and appoint a trusted individual to make healthcare decisions on their behalf if they become unable to do so themselves. By documenting their wishes in advance, aging parents can ensure that their healthcare preferences are known and respected by caregivers and healthcare providers, and that their end-of-life care is guided by their values, beliefs, and preferences. Advance directives and healthcare proxies empower aging parents to make informed decisions about their healthcare and end-of-life care, giving them a sense of control and autonomy as they age.

9.3 Providing Comfort and Palliative Care

Providing comfort and palliative care is a crucial aspect of end-of-life care and decision-making when caring for aging parents. Palliative care focuses on relieving symptoms and improving the quality of life for individuals with serious illness or nearing the end of life, regardless of prognosis. It emphasizes holistic care that addresses physical, emotional, social, and spiritual needs, aiming to maximize comfort, dignity, and quality of life for both patients and their families.

1. Importance of Comfort and Palliative Care: Providing comfort and palliative care is essential for aging parents who are facing serious illness or nearing the end of life. Palliative care focuses on alleviating

symptoms such as pain, shortness of breath, fatigue, nausea, and anxiety, which can significantly impact quality of life and well-being. By addressing these symptoms and providing holistic support, palliative care helps improve the overall comfort, dignity, and quality of life for aging parents and their families. Palliative care also emphasizes open and honest communication, shared decision-making, and advance care planning, enabling aging parents to make informed decisions about their healthcare and end-of-life care preferences.

2. Principles and Goals of Palliative Care: Palliative care is guided by several key principles and goals, including:

> a. Holistic Care: Palliative care addresses the physical, emotional, social, and spiritual needs of patients and their families, recognizing the interconnectedness of these domains and their impact on overall well-being.

> b. Symptom Management: Palliative care focuses on relieving symptoms and managing side effects of illness and treatment, such as pain, nausea, fatigue, and shortness of breath, to improve comfort and quality of life.

> c. Communication and Shared Decision-Making: Palliative care emphasizes open and honest communication between patients, families, and healthcare providers, facilitating shared decision-making and informed choices about healthcare and end-of-life care preferences.

d. Advance Care Planning: Palliative care encourages advance care planning, including the completion of advance directives and discussions about goals of care, preferences for medical treatment, and end-of-life wishes.

e. Supportive Care: Palliative care provides emotional, psychosocial, and spiritual support to patients and families, helping them cope with the challenges of serious illness and end-of-life care decisions.

f. Quality of Life: The primary goal of palliative care is to maximize comfort, dignity, and quality of life for patients and families, focusing on what matters most to the individual and their loved ones.

3. Integrating Palliative Care into End-of-Life Care Planning: Integrating palliative care into end-of-life care planning involves several key steps, including:

a. Assessment and Symptom Management: Conducting a comprehensive assessment of aging parents' symptoms and addressing any issues that may impact their comfort and quality of life, such as pain, nausea, fatigue, and shortness of breath. This may involve medication management, complementary therapies, and supportive interventions to alleviate symptoms and improve well-being.

b. Advance Care Planning: Engaging aging parents in discussions about their goals of care, preferences for medical treatment, and end-of-life wishes, and documenting these preferences in advance directives, such as living wills and healthcare proxies. Advance care planning ensures that aging parents' wishes are known and respected by caregivers and healthcare providers, and that their end-of-life care is guided by their values, beliefs, and preferences.

c. Communication and Shared Decision-Making: Facilitating open and honest communication between aging parents, family members, and healthcare providers, and encouraging shared decision-making and collaboration in healthcare and end-of-life care decisions. This may involve discussing treatment options, prognosis, and goals of care, and exploring how interventions align with aging parents' preferences and values.

d. Psychosocial and Spiritual Support: Providing emotional, psychosocial, and spiritual support to aging parents and their families, helping them cope with the emotional and existential challenges of serious illness and end-of-life care. This may involve counseling, support groups, spiritual care, and other supportive services to address the psychological and spiritual needs of patients and families.

e. Family Caregiver Support: Offering support and resources to family caregivers who play a crucial role in providing care and support to aging parents. This may involve respite care, caregiver education and training, and assistance with navigating the healthcare system and accessing supportive services.

f. Continuity of Care: Ensuring continuity of care for aging parents by coordinating care across settings and providers, including hospitals, nursing homes, hospice programs, and community-based services. This may involve care coordination, case management, and regular communication between healthcare providers to ensure that aging parents' needs are met and that care is delivered in a coordinated and seamless manner.

4. Providing Comfort Measures and Supportive Interventions: Providing comfort measures and supportive interventions is essential for meeting the physical, emotional, social, and spiritual needs of aging parents receiving palliative care. Some key comfort measures and supportive interventions include:

a. Pain Management: Ensuring that aging parents receive adequate pain relief through medication management, non-pharmacological interventions, and complementary therapies, such as massage, acupuncture, and relaxation techniques.

b. Symptom Management: Addressing other symptoms that may impact aging parents' comfort and quality of life, such as nausea, fatigue, shortness of breath, and anxiety, through medication management, supportive care, and symptom-specific interventions.

c. Emotional Support: Providing emotional support to aging parents and their families, helping them cope with the psychological and existential challenges of serious illness and end-of-life care. This may involve counseling, psychotherapy, support groups, and other interventions to address feelings of sadness, fear, anger, and grief.

d. Social Support: Facilitating social connections and engagement for aging parents, helping them maintain relationships with family and friends, participate in meaningful activities, and preserve their sense of identity and purpose. This may involve visits from loved ones, participation in social activities, and connection to community-based services and resources.

e. Spiritual Care: Offering spiritual care and support to aging parents and their families, helping them find meaning, purpose, and comfort in their beliefs and values. This may involve spiritual counseling, prayer, meditation, and connection to religious or spiritual communities and practices.

5. Navigating Difficult Decisions and End-of-Life Transitions: Navigating difficult decisions and end-of-life transitions can be emotionally challenging for aging parents and their families, especially as illness progresses and care needs increase. Some key strategies for navigating these challenges include:

a. Open and Honest Communication: Encouraging open and honest communication between aging parents, family members, and healthcare providers, and fostering shared decision-making and collaboration in end-of-life care decisions.

b. Respecting Autonomy and Dignity: Respecting aging parents' autonomy and dignity by honoring their wishes and preferences for medical treatment and end-of-life care, and involving them in decision-making to the extent possible given their cognitive and functional status.

c. Providing Compassionate Care: Providing compassionate care and support to aging parents and their families throughout the end-of-life care journey, offering comfort, reassurance, and companionship during times of illness, transition, and loss.

d. Anticipatory Guidance: Providing anticipatory guidance and support to aging parents and their families as they navigate the challenges of serious illness and end-of-life care, including discussions about prognosis, goals of care, and advance care planning.

e. Bereavement Support: Offering bereavement support and counseling to family members and caregivers following the death of an aging parent, helping them cope with grief, loss, and adjustment to life without their loved one.

Providing comfort and palliative care is essential for meeting the physical, emotional, social, and spiritual needs of aging parents as they face serious illness or approach the end of life. Palliative care focuses on relieving symptoms, improving quality of life, and supporting aging parents and their families through the challenges of serious illness and end-of-life care decisions. By integrating palliative care into end-of-life care planning, addressing the holistic needs of aging parents, and providing compassionate care and support throughout the end-of-life care journey, families can ensure that aging parents receive the care and comfort they need to live their final days with dignity, peace, and quality of life.

9.4 Coping with Grief and Loss

Coping with grief and loss is an inevitable part of the end-of-life care journey when caring for aging parents. As aging parents approach the end of life, caregivers and family members often experience a range of emotions, including sadness, grief, anger, guilt, and anxiety. Coping with these emotions can be challenging, but it is essential for caregivers and family members to find healthy ways to process their grief and navigate the grieving process effectively. This section reiterates some of what was earlier mentioned in chapter 5.

1. Understand the Grieving Process: The grieving process is a natural and normal response to loss, encompassing a range of emotions, thoughts, and behaviors that individuals may experience following the death of a loved one. The grieving process is often described in stages, although it is important to recognize that grief is unique to each individual and may not follow a linear progression. Some common stages of grief include:

> a. Shock and Denial: Initially, individuals may feel shocked or numb in response to the death of a loved one, and may have difficulty accepting the reality of the loss.

b. Anger and Guilt: As the reality of the loss sets in, individuals may experience feelings of anger, resentment, or guilt, directed towards themselves, others, or the deceased.

c. Sadness and Depression: Grief often involves profound feelings of sadness, emptiness, and despair, as individuals come to terms with the reality of the loss and the impact it has on their lives.

d. Acceptance and Healing: Over time, individuals may gradually come to accept the reality of the loss and find ways to adjust to life without their loved one, although the pain of the loss may never fully disappear.

2. Challenges of Coping with Grief and Loss When Caring for Aging Parents: Coping with grief and loss when caring for aging parents presents unique challenges and stressors for caregivers and family members. Some of these challenges may include:

a. Anticipatory Grief: Caregivers and family members may experience anticipatory grief as they anticipate the death of an aging parent, particularly if the parent has a serious illness or declining health. Anticipatory grief can be intense and overwhelming, and may involve feelings of sadness, anxiety, and uncertainty about the future.

b. Role Reversal and Caregiver Stress: Caring for an aging parent at the end of life often involves significant role reversal, as adult children assume the role of caregivers and provide physical, emotional, and practical support to their parents. This role reversal can be emotionally taxing and may lead to feelings of stress, burnout, and caregiver burden.

c. Complicated Family Dynamics: Coping with grief and loss within the family unit can be complicated by existing family dynamics, conflicts, and unresolved issues. Differences in coping styles, communication patterns, and expectations among family members may contribute to tension and conflict during the grieving process.

d. Practical and Financial Concerns: In addition to emotional challenges, caregivers and family members may face practical and financial concerns related to end-of-life care, funeral arrangements, and estate matters. These practical concerns can add to the stress and burden of coping with grief and loss.

3. Strategies for Coping with Grief and Loss When Caring for Aging Parents: Coping with grief and loss when caring for aging parents requires self-awareness, self-care, and support from others. Some strategies for coping with grief and loss include:

a. Acknowledge and Validate Feelings: Allow yourself to feel and express a range of emotions, including sadness, anger, guilt, and fear. Acknowledge that grief is a natural and normal response to loss, and validate your feelings without judgment or self-criticism.

b. Seek Support from Others: Reach out to friends, family members, support groups, or mental health professionals for emotional support and guidance. Sharing your thoughts and feelings with others who have experienced similar losses can provide comfort, validation, and perspective.

c. Practice Self-Care: Take care of your physical, emotional, and spiritual well-being by engaging in self-care activities that promote relaxation, stress reduction, and overall well-being. This may include exercise, meditation, yoga, hobbies, or spending time in nature.

d. Set Boundaries and Prioritize Self-Care: Establish boundaries with yourself and others to protect your emotional and physical well-being. Prioritize self-care activities and give yourself permission to say no to additional responsibilities or commitments that may exacerbate stress and overwhelm.

e. Maintain Open Communication: Foster open and honest communication with family members and loved ones about your thoughts, feelings, and needs during the grieving process. Share your experiences, listen to others' perspectives, and work together to navigate the challenges of grief and loss as a family.

f. Seek Professional Help if Needed: If you are struggling to cope with grief and loss on your own, consider seeking support from a mental health professional, such as a therapist or grief counselor. A trained professional can offer guidance, support, and coping strategies to help you navigate the grieving process effectively.

g. Honor Your Loved One's Memory: Find meaningful ways to honor your aging parent's memory and legacy, such as creating a memory book or scrapbook, planting a memorial garden, participating in a memorial service or tribute, or engaging in activities that were meaningful to your loved one.

h. Practice Self-Compassion and Patience: Be gentle and patient with yourself as you navigate the ups and downs of grief and loss. Practice self-compassion by offering yourself kindness, understanding, and acceptance during difficult times, and remind yourself that healing takes time and effort.

4. Supporting Others Through Grief and Loss: Supporting others through grief and loss involves providing empathy, validation, and practical support to help them navigate the grieving process effectively. Some ways to support others through grief and loss include:

a. Listen with Empathy: Listen attentively to the person's thoughts, feelings, and experiences without judgment or interruption. Offer empathy, validation, and validation, and validate their feelings and experiences.

b. Offer Practical Support: Offer practical support to help the person with daily tasks, responsibilities, and errands, such as meal preparation, household chores, childcare, or transportation.

c. Provide Emotional Support: Provide emotional support by offering a listening ear, a shoulder to cry on, or a comforting presence during difficult times. Offer words of encouragement, validation, and reassurance to help the person feel supported and understood.

d. Respect Their Needs and Boundaries: Respect the person's needs and boundaries by honoring their preferences for privacy, space, and solitude when needed. Allow the person to express their grief in their own way and at their own pace, without pressure or judgment.

e. Encourage Self-Care: Encourage the person to engage in self-care activities that promote relaxation, stress reduction, and overall well-being, such as exercise, meditation, hobbies, or spending time with loved ones.

f. Provide Resources and Referrals: Provide information about grief support groups, counseling services, and other resources that may be helpful for the person as they navigate the grieving process. Offer to accompany them to appointments or meetings if needed.

Coping with grief and loss when caring for aging parents is a complex and challenging process that requires self-awareness, self-care, and support from others. By acknowledging and validating your feelings, seeking support from friends, family, and professionals, practicing self-care, and supporting others through their grief and loss, you can navigate the grieving process effectively and find healing and meaning in the midst of loss. Remember that grief is a natural and normal response to loss, and that healing takes time and effort. By honoring your loved one's memory and legacy, you can find solace and comfort in the midst of grief, and carry their love and presence with you as you continue on your own journey of healing and growth.

Chapter 10: Nurturing Relationships Across Generations

10.1 Fostering Intergenerational Connections

Fostering Intergenerational Connections is a crucial aspect of nurturing relationships across generations, promoting understanding, empathy, and mutual respect between individuals of different age groups. Intergenerational connections involve interactions, activities, and experiences that bridge the gap between generations, fostering meaningful relationships, shared experiences, and a sense of belonging and connection within families and communities.

Intergenerational connections refer to interactions, relationships, and exchanges between individuals of different age groups, particularly between younger and older generations, that promote understanding, empathy, and mutual support. Intergenerational connections encompass a wide range of activities and experiences, including family gatherings, shared hobbies and interests, community service projects, mentorship programs, and intergenerational learning initiatives.

Importance of Fostering Intergenerational Connections

1. Promoting Understanding and Empathy: Intergenerational connections promote understanding and empathy between individuals of different age groups by fostering communication,

shared experiences, and mutual respect, breaking down stereotypes and generational barriers.

2. Passing on Wisdom and Experience: Intergenerational connections provide opportunities for older generations to pass on wisdom, knowledge, and life experience to younger generations, serving as mentors, role models, and sources of guidance and inspiration.

3. Building Stronger Families and Communities: Intergenerational connections strengthen families and communities by fostering a sense of belonging, connection, and shared identity across generations, and promoting collaboration, cooperation, and support among individuals of all ages.

4. Addressing Social Isolation and Loneliness: Intergenerational connections reduce social isolation and loneliness for individuals of all ages by providing opportunities for socialization, companionship, and engagement with others, particularly for older adults who may be at risk of isolation.

5. Enhancing Emotional Well-being: Intergenerational connections enhance emotional well-being for individuals of all ages by providing social support, validation, and companionship, and fostering a sense of purpose, belonging, and fulfillment in relationships with others.

6. Promoting Lifelong Learning and Growth: Intergenerational connections promote lifelong learning and growth by facilitating the exchange of knowledge, skills, and perspectives across generations,

and fostering curiosity, creativity, and intellectual stimulation in individuals of all ages.

Examples of Activities and Initiatives for Fostering Intergenerational Connections

1. Family Gatherings and Traditions: Organize family gatherings, celebrations, and traditions that bring together members of different generations to share stories, experiences, and memories, and strengthen family bonds and connections.

2. Intergenerational Learning Programs: Participate in intergenerational learning programs and initiatives that bring together children, youth, and older adults to engage in educational activities, such as reading programs, art classes, and science and engineering projects, and promote learning and skill development across generations.

3. Volunteer and Community Service Projects: Engage in volunteer and community service projects that involve individuals of different ages working together to address community needs, such as environmental clean-up efforts, food drives, and intergenerational mentorship programs.

4. Mentorship and Coaching Programs: Participate in mentorship and coaching programs that pair older adults with younger individuals to provide guidance, support, and encouragement in areas such as career development, academic success, and personal growth.

5. Intergenerational Housing and Living Arrangements: Explore intergenerational housing and living arrangements that bring together individuals of different ages to live and collaborate in shared spaces, fostering mutual support, companionship, and interdependence.

6. Cultural and Recreational Activities: Participate in cultural and recreational activities that appeal to individuals of all ages, such as music concerts, art exhibits, theater performances, and outdoor adventures, and provide opportunities for intergenerational bonding and enjoyment.

7. Storytelling and Oral History Projects: Engage in storytelling and oral history projects that involve individuals of different generations sharing and preserving personal stories, family histories, and cultural traditions, and passing on wisdom and heritage to future generations.

8. Technology and Digital Literacy Programs: Participate in technology and digital literacy programs that bring together younger and older individuals to learn and explore new technologies, such as computers, smartphones, and social media platforms, and bridge the digital divide between generations.

Strategies for Nurturing Relationships Across Generations

1. Promote Open Communication: Encourage open communication and dialogue between individuals of different age groups, fostering active listening, respect, and understanding of diverse perspectives and experiences.

2. Create Shared Experiences: Create opportunities for shared experiences and activities that bring together individuals of different generations, fostering connections, memories, and bonds that transcend age differences.

3. Encourage Mutual Learning and Growth: Encourage mutual learning and growth by creating environments that value the contributions and perspectives of individuals of all ages, and promote collaboration, mentorship, and peer support across generations.

4. Respect Differences and Diversity: Respect differences and diversity among individuals of different age groups, including cultural backgrounds, beliefs, and preferences, and foster an inclusive and accepting environment that celebrates the richness of intergenerational relationships.

5. Provide Support and Resources: Provide support and resources for individuals and families to engage in intergenerational activities and initiatives, including access to educational programs, community resources, and intergenerational learning opportunities.

6. Lead by Example: Lead by example in fostering intergenerational connections and relationships, demonstrating empathy, respect, and appreciation for individuals of all ages, and promoting the value of intergenerational collaboration and cooperation in families and communities.

7. Advocate for Intergenerational Initiatives: Advocate for intergenerational initiatives and policies that support and promote

intergenerational connections and relationships, and address barriers and challenges to intergenerational collaboration and engagement in society.

Benefits of Embracing Intergenerational Connections

1. Enhanced Social and Emotional Well-being: Embracing intergenerational connections enhances social and emotional well-being for individuals of all ages by providing opportunities for connection, companionship, and support across generations.

2. Promotion of Understanding and Empathy: Intergenerational connections promote understanding and empathy between individuals of different age groups, fostering respect, appreciation, and acceptance of diverse perspectives and experiences.

3. Building Stronger Families and Communities: Intergenerational connections strengthen families and communities by fostering a sense of belonging, connection, and shared identity across generations, and promoting cooperation, collaboration, and mutual support.

4. Promotion of Lifelong Learning and Growth: Intergenerational connections promote lifelong learning and growth by facilitating the exchange of knowledge, skills, and experiences across generations, and fostering curiosity, creativity, and intellectual stimulation in individuals of all ages.

5. Addressing Social Isolation and Loneliness: Intergenerational connections reduce social isolation and loneliness for individuals of

all ages by providing opportunities for socialization, companionship, and engagement with others, particularly for older adults who may be at risk of isolation.

Fostering intergenerational connections is essential for nurturing relationships across generations, promoting understanding, empathy, and mutual respect between individuals of different age groups, and building stronger families and communities. By embracing intergenerational connections and engaging in activities and initiatives that bring together individuals of all ages, we can create environments that value the contributions and perspectives of individuals of all ages, and promote collaboration, cooperation, and support across generations, ultimately enhancing social and emotional well-being for individuals and society as a whole.

10.2 Passing Down Family Traditions and Values

Passing Down Family Traditions and Values is a fundamental aspect of nurturing relationships across generations, preserving cultural heritage, and strengthening family bonds. Family traditions and values serve as the cornerstone of identity, belonging, and connection within families, providing a sense of continuity, shared history, and purpose across generations.

Family traditions are customs, rituals, and practices that are passed down from generation to generation within a family, often involving shared activities, celebrations, and ceremonies that hold significance and meaning for family members. Family values are principles, beliefs, and ideals that guide the behavior, decisions, and interactions of family members, shaping the culture, identity, and legacy of the family over time.

Importance of Passing Down Family Traditions and Values

1. Preserving Cultural Heritage: Passing down family traditions and values preserves cultural heritage and identity, ensuring that customs, beliefs, and practices are transmitted from one generation to the next, and maintaining a connection to the past and ancestral roots.

2. Strengthening Family Bonds: Family traditions and values strengthen family bonds and relationships by providing opportunities for shared experiences, connection, and belonging among family members, and fostering a sense of unity, cohesion, and support within the family unit.

3. Instilling Identity and Purpose: Family traditions and values instill a sense of identity and purpose in individuals by providing a framework for understanding one's place within the family and society, and reinforcing core principles and ideals that guide behavior and decision-making.

4. Promoting Intergenerational Communication: Passing down family traditions and values promotes intergenerational communication and dialogue between older and younger family members, facilitating the exchange of stories, memories, and wisdom, and fostering understanding, empathy, and connection across generations.

5. Building Resilience and Adaptability: Family traditions and values build resilience and adaptability in individuals and families by providing a sense of stability, continuity, and belonging in times of change or adversity, and serving as a source of strength and support during challenging times.

6. Transmitting Life Lessons and Wisdom: Family traditions and values transmit life lessons, wisdom, and moral teachings from one generation to the next, providing guidance, inspiration, and perspective on navigating life's challenges and opportunities.

Examples of Family Traditions and Values

1. Holiday Celebrations: Holiday celebrations such as Thanksgiving, Christmas, and Hanukkah involve family gatherings, feasts, and rituals that hold special significance and meaning for family members, reinforcing values of gratitude, generosity, and togetherness.

2. Cultural Practices: Cultural practices such as language, cuisine, music, and dance are passed down through generations, preserving cultural identity and heritage, and fostering a sense of pride and belonging in one's cultural heritage.

3. Family Rituals: Family rituals such as weekly dinners, bedtime stories, and birthday traditions provide opportunities for connection, bonding, and reflection among family members, and reinforce values of love, respect, and family unity.

4. Religious Observances: Religious observances such as attending religious services at places of worship, participating in religious festivals, and observing religious rituals and customs transmit religious beliefs, values, and traditions from one generation to the next, and provide a spiritual foundation for individuals and families.

5. Ethical Principles: Ethical principles such as honesty, integrity, and compassion are instilled through family values and teachings, guiding moral behavior and decision-making in individuals and families, and promoting ethical conduct and social responsibility.

6. Generational Stories and Wisdom: Generational stories, anecdotes, and wisdom passed down through oral tradition convey lessons learned, experiences shared, and values upheld by previous generations, providing inspiration, guidance, and perspective for younger family members.

Strategies for Preserving and Transmitting Family Traditions and Values

1. Document Family History: Document family history, stories, and traditions through oral interviews, written accounts, photographs, and videos, preserving memories and experiences for future generations to learn from and appreciate.

2. Celebrate Family Milestones: Celebrate family milestones and achievements such as births, weddings, graduations, and anniversaries with meaningful rituals and traditions that reinforce family values and strengthen bonds among family members.

3. Pass on Skills and Knowledge: Pass on skills, knowledge, and expertise through hands-on experiences, mentorship, and apprenticeship, teaching younger family members practical skills, hobbies, and crafts that have been passed down through generations.

4. Create Family Traditions: Create new family traditions and rituals that reflect the values, interests, and identities of current family members, incorporating elements of culture, religion, and personal significance to create meaningful experiences and connections.

5. Engage in Intergenerational Activities: Engage in intergenerational activities and experiences that bring together individuals of different ages to learn, collaborate, and bond, such as cooking together, gardening, storytelling, and community service projects.

6. Lead by Example: Lead by example in embodying and practicing family values and traditions in everyday life, demonstrating integrity, kindness, and respect in interactions with others, and serving as role models for younger family members to emulate.

7. Facilitate Open Communication: Facilitate open communication and dialogue within the family to discuss and share stories, memories, and experiences related to family traditions and values, encouraging active listening, empathy, and understanding among family members.

8. Embrace Change and Adaptability: Embrace change and adaptability in family traditions and values, recognizing that

traditions may evolve over time to reflect changing circumstances, lifestyles, and cultural influences, while maintaining core values and principles that anchor the family identity and legacy.

Benefits of Embracing and Perpetuating Family Heritage

1. Strengthened Family Bonds: Embracing and perpetuating family heritage strengthens family bonds and relationships by providing a sense of continuity, connection, and shared identity across generations.

2. Preservation of Cultural Heritage: Embracing and perpetuating family heritage preserves cultural heritage and identity, ensuring that customs, beliefs, and practices are passed down and cherished by future generations.

3. Transmission of Values and Wisdom: Embracing and perpetuating family heritage transmit values, wisdom, and life lessons from one generation to the next, providing guidance, inspiration, and perspective on navigating life's challenges and opportunities.

4. Enhanced Sense of Belonging: Embracing and perpetuating family heritage fosters a sense of belonging and rootedness in individuals and families, providing a sense of identity, purpose, and connection to one's roots and ancestral lineage.

5. Promotion of Intergenerational Communication: Embracing and perpetuating family heritage promotes intergenerational communication and understanding, facilitating the exchange of stories, memories, and experiences between older and younger

family members, and fostering empathy, respect, and appreciation for diverse perspectives and experiences.

Passing down family traditions and values is essential for nurturing relationships across generations, preserving cultural heritage, and strengthening family bonds. By embracing and perpetuating family heritage, individuals and families can preserve cherished customs, beliefs, and practices, and transmit values, wisdom, and life lessons from one generation to the next, fostering a sense of connection, continuity, and belonging within families and communities.

10.3 Planning for Your Own Aging Journey

Planning for Your Own Aging Journey is a proactive approach to preparing for the inevitable changes and challenges that come with aging. It involves making decisions and arrangements to ensure that one's future needs and preferences are met, while also considering the impact of these decisions on family members and loved ones. Planning for one's own aging journey is not only a practical step towards ensuring a comfortable and fulfilling later life but also a way to nurture relationships across generations by relieving potential burdens on family members and promoting open communication about aging-related topics.

Aging planning is the process of making decisions and arrangements to prepare for the changes and challenges that come with aging, including financial, legal, healthcare, and lifestyle considerations. Aging planning encompasses a wide range of topics and areas of life, including retirement planning, healthcare planning, long-term care planning, estate planning, and end-of-life planning.

Importance of Planning for Your Own Aging Journey

1. Empowerment and Control: Planning for one's own aging journey empowers individuals to make informed decisions about their future care, finances, and lifestyle preferences, and maintain a sense of control and autonomy over their lives as they age.

2. Relieving Burdens on Family Members: Aging planning relieves potential burdens on family members and loved ones by clearly outlining one's wishes and preferences for future care, reducing uncertainty and stress for family caregivers and decision-makers.

3. Ensuring Quality of Life: Aging planning ensures that individuals can maintain a high quality of life as they age by anticipating and addressing potential challenges and needs, such as healthcare, housing, and support services, and making arrangements to meet those needs.

4. Promoting Open Communication: Aging planning promotes open communication and dialogue among family members about aging-related topics, including end-of-life wishes, caregiving roles, and financial responsibilities, fostering understanding, empathy, and support within the family unit.

5. Protecting Assets and Legacy: Aging planning protects assets and legacy by implementing strategies to manage and preserve wealth, plan for potential long-term care expenses, and distribute assets

according to one's wishes through estate planning and legal arrangements.

6. Reducing Stress and Anxiety: Aging planning reduces stress and anxiety about the future by providing peace of mind and reassurance that one's needs and preferences will be addressed, and potential challenges will be managed effectively through proactive planning and preparation.

Key Considerations and Decisions in Aging Planning

1. Financial Planning: Evaluate financial resources, retirement savings, and income sources to ensure sufficient funds are available to cover living expenses, healthcare costs, and long-term care needs in retirement.

2. Healthcare Planning: Consider healthcare needs and preferences, including medical care, long-term care options, advance care planning, and end-of-life care decisions, and make arrangements to ensure access to quality healthcare services.

3. Legal Planning: Review and update legal documents such as wills, trusts, powers of attorney, and advance directives to ensure they accurately reflect one's wishes and preferences for asset distribution, decision-making authority, and medical treatment.

4. Housing and Lifestyle Planning: Evaluate housing options and lifestyle preferences for aging in place, downsizing, or transitioning to assisted living or other supportive environments that meet changing needs and preferences.

5. Social Support and Caregiving Planning: Identify potential sources of social support and caregiving assistance from family members, friends, community services, and professional caregivers, and make arrangements for ongoing care and support as needed.

6. End-of-Life Planning: Discuss end-of-life wishes and preferences for funeral arrangements, organ donation, and legacy planning with loved ones, and document these preferences in advance directives and other legal documents.

7. Legacy Planning: Consider legacy planning goals and objectives for passing on values, beliefs, and assets to future generations, and develop strategies for preserving and transferring wealth and assets in accordance with one's wishes.

Strategies for Effective Aging Planning

1. Start Early: Start the aging planning process early to allow time for thorough assessment, decision-making, and implementation of strategies to address future needs and preferences.

2. Seek Professional Guidance: Consult with financial advisors, estate planners, elder law attorneys, healthcare professionals, and other experts to obtain guidance and assistance in navigating complex aging planning issues and making informed decisions.

3. Involve Family Members: Involve family members and loved ones in the aging planning process to ensure that their concerns, preferences, and perspectives are taken into account, and foster open communication and collaboration in decision-making.

4. Review and Update Plans Regularly: Review and update aging plans regularly to reflect changes in personal circumstances, health status, financial resources, and legal requirements, and ensure that plans remain relevant and effective over time.

5. Educate Yourself: Educate yourself about aging-related topics, including healthcare options, legal rights, financial planning strategies, and end-of-life issues, to make informed decisions and advocate for your own needs and preferences.

6. Be Flexible and Adaptable: Be flexible and adaptable in your aging planning approach, recognizing that circumstances may change, and unexpected challenges may arise, requiring adjustments to plans and strategies along the way.

7. Communicate Openly and Honestly: Communicate openly and honestly with family members and loved ones about aging planning decisions, concerns, and wishes, and encourage dialogue and collaboration in addressing shared goals and priorities.

Benefits of Proactive Aging Planning

1. Peace of Mind: Proactive aging planning provides peace of mind and reassurance that one's needs and preferences will be addressed, and potential challenges will be managed effectively, reducing stress and anxiety about the future.

2. Empowerment and Autonomy: Proactive aging planning empowers individuals to make informed decisions about their

future care, finances, and lifestyle preferences, and maintain a sense of control and autonomy over their lives as they age.

3. Support for Family Members: Proactive aging planning supports family members and loved ones by relieving potential burdens and uncertainties about caregiving roles, financial responsibilities, and end-of-life decisions, and promoting open communication and collaboration in addressing aging-related issues.

4. Preservation of Dignity and Independence: Proactive aging planning preserves dignity and independence by allowing individuals to make choices and decisions about their future care, housing, and lifestyle preferences, and maintain control over important aspects of their lives as they age.

5. Protection of Assets and Legacy: Proactive aging planning protects assets and legacy by implementing strategies to manage and preserve wealth, plan for potential long-term care expenses, and distribute assets according to one's wishes through estate planning and legal arrangements.

6. Enhanced Quality of Life: Proactive aging planning enhances the quality of life for individuals as they age by ensuring access to necessary care, support, and resources, and promoting well-being, fulfillment, and dignity in later life.

Planning for one's own aging journey is a proactive and empowering approach to preparing for the changes and challenges that come with aging. By making informed decisions and arrangements to address future needs and preferences, individuals can ensure a comfortable and fulfilling later life while also relieving potential burdens on family members and promoting open communication and collaboration in addressing aging-related issues. Proactive aging planning provides peace of mind, empowers individuals to maintain control and autonomy over their lives, and supports family members and loved ones in navigating the complexities of aging with dignity and grace.

10.4 Embracing the Legacy of Love and Care

"Embracing the Legacy of Love and Care" is a profound acknowledgment of the enduring impact that acts of love and care have on individuals and families across generations. It encompasses recognizing, honoring, and preserving the legacy of compassion, support, and connection passed down from one generation to the next, and embodying these values in our relationships and interactions with others. Embracing the legacy of love and care involves cherishing memories, honoring the contributions of past generations, and fostering a culture of empathy, kindness, and generosity within families and communities.

The legacy of love and care refers to the enduring impact of acts of kindness, compassion, and support passed down from one generation to the next, shaping family relationships, values, and traditions over time. The legacy of love and care encompasses a wide range of behaviors, attitudes, and experiences, including expressions of affection, acts of service, emotional support, and nurturing relationships within families and communities.

Importance of Embracing the Legacy of Love and Care

1. Continuity and Connection: Embracing the legacy of love and care fosters continuity and connection across generations by honoring the contributions and sacrifices of past generations and reinforcing the bonds of love and kinship that unite family members.

2. Cultivation of Empathy and Compassion: Embracing the legacy of love and care cultivates empathy and compassion in individuals by modeling selfless acts of kindness, generosity, and support within families and communities, and fostering a culture of caring and empathy for others.

3. Preservation of Family Heritage: Embracing the legacy of love and care preserves family heritage and traditions by passing down values, beliefs, and practices that reflect the importance of love, compassion, and mutual support in nurturing strong and resilient family relationships.

4. Promotion of Well-being and Resilience: Embracing the legacy of love and care promotes well-being and resilience in individuals and families by providing a foundation of love, acceptance, and support that fosters emotional security, self-esteem, and positive relationships with others.

5. Inspiration for Future Generations: Embracing the legacy of love and care inspires future generations to carry forward the values and principles of compassion, kindness, and generosity in their own lives, ensuring that the legacy of love and care continues to thrive and evolve over time.

6. Healing and Reconciliation: Embracing the legacy of love and care can facilitate healing and reconciliation within families by fostering forgiveness, understanding, and acceptance of past hurts and conflicts, and promoting a sense of unity, harmony, and belonging among family members.

Examples of Embracing the Legacy of Love and Care

1. Expressions of Affection: Embracing the legacy of love and care involves expressing affection and appreciation for family members through hugs, kisses, and words of encouragement, affirming the value and importance of love and connection in family relationships.

2. Acts of Service: Embracing the legacy of love and care includes performing acts of service and kindness for others, such as helping with household chores, running errands, or providing emotional support during difficult times, demonstrating a commitment to supporting and nurturing others.

3. Quality Time Together: Embracing the legacy of love and care entails spending quality time together as a family, engaging in shared activities, conversations, and experiences that strengthen bonds and create lasting memories of love and connection.

4. Supportive Relationships: Embracing the legacy of love and care involves cultivating supportive relationships within families, characterized by trust, empathy, and mutual respect, and providing a safe and nurturing environment where individuals can thrive and grow.

5. Generosity and Giving: Embracing the legacy of love and care encompasses acts of generosity and giving to others in need, whether through charitable donations, volunteer work, or acts of kindness and compassion towards those facing adversity, reflecting a commitment to making a positive difference in the lives of others.

6. Honoring Family Traditions: Embracing the legacy of love and care includes honoring family traditions and customs that celebrate love, unity, and connection, such as family gatherings, holiday celebrations, and rituals that reinforce the importance of family bonds and relationships.

Strategies for Nurturing and Preserving the Legacy of Love and Care

1. Lead by Example: Lead by example in embodying the values of love, compassion, and care in your own actions and interactions with others, demonstrating kindness, empathy, and generosity in your relationships with family members and loved ones.

2. Share Family Stories and Memories: Share family stories, memories, and traditions that highlight acts of love and care passed down through generations, preserving the legacy of compassion and connection within the family and inspiring future generations to carry forward these values.

3. Create Meaningful Rituals and Traditions: Create meaningful rituals and traditions that honor the legacy of love and care within your family, such as annual family reunions, special celebrations, or acts of service and kindness that bring family members together and reinforce the importance of love and connection.

4. Encourage Open Communication: Encourage open communication and dialogue within your family about the importance of love, compassion, and support in nurturing strong and resilient relationships, and create a safe and supportive environment where family members feel comfortable expressing their feelings and needs.

5. Provide Emotional Support: Provide emotional support and encouragement to family members during difficult times, offering a listening ear, words of comfort, and practical assistance as needed, and demonstrating a commitment to being there for each other through thick and thin.

6. Celebrate Achievements and Milestones: Celebrate achievements and milestones within your family, such as graduations, weddings, and anniversaries, with expressions of love and support that reinforce the bonds of family and the importance of celebrating life's joys together.

7. Practice Forgiveness and Understanding: Practice forgiveness and understanding in your relationships with family members, acknowledging and addressing past hurts and conflicts with empathy and compassion, and working towards reconciliation and healing within the family unit.

Benefits of Embracing the Legacy of Love and Care

1. Strengthened Family Bonds: Embracing the legacy of love and care strengthens family bonds and relationships by fostering a culture of empathy, kindness, and support within families, and promoting unity, harmony, and resilience in times of need.

2. Promotion of Emotional Well-being: Embracing the legacy of love and care promotes emotional well-being and fulfillment in individuals and families by providing a foundation of love, acceptance, and support that nurtures self-esteem and positive relationships with others.

3. Inspiration for Future Generations: Embracing the legacy of love and care inspires future generations to carry forward the values and principles of compassion, kindness, and generosity in their lives, ensuring that the legacy of love and care continues to thrive and evolve over time.

4. Cultivation of Empathy and Compassion: Embracing the legacy of love and care cultivates empathy and compassion in individuals by modeling selfless acts of kindness, generosity, and support within families and communities, and fostering a culture of caring for others.

5. Enhanced Sense of Connection and Belonging: Embracing the legacy of love and care fosters a sense of connection and belonging within families by honoring the contributions and sacrifices of past generations and reinforcing the bonds of love and kinship that unite family members.

Embracing the legacy of love and care is a transformative journey of recognizing, honoring, and preserving the enduring impact of acts of kindness, compassion, and support passed down through generations. By cherishing memories, honoring the contributions of past generations, and embodying these values in our relationships and interactions with others, we can nurture strong and resilient family bonds, promote empathy and compassion within families and communities, and inspire future generations to carry forward the legacy of love and care for generations to come.